The Ultimate Guide to a Beautiful Smile

Everything You Need to Know Before Getting Braces or Invisalign

Dr. Matthew R. Wirig

DEDICATION

To my beautiful wife and amazing children. You inspire me.

You can set up your FREE exam and X-Rays ($300 value) at our Henderson or Las Vegas locations by calling (702) 848-4585!

Get your free Orthodontic Decision-Making Kit! Just go to http://UltimateSmileGuide.com. Your kit includes:

- Our report, "The Caring Parent's Guide To Orthodontics: Five Factors To Know Before Getting Braces or Invisalign"

- A downloadable recording of Dr. Wirig on Business Innovators Radio called "Specialization and Technology: How To Get The Fastest, Most Comfortable Orthodontic Treatment Available"

- A digital copy of this book

Go to http://UltimateSmileGuide.com!

CONTENTS

FOREWORD

Should you see an orthodontist? How do you know? It can be confusing to figure it all out. Does my child really need braces? How much will it cost? How long will the braces need to stay on? Will it hurt? What foods can my child eat while wearing braces?

In this guide, I'll cover some of the questions you, as a parent, may have about orthodontics and your child's health. If you are interested in getting braces for yourself, much of the information in this book will be relevant to you as well.

Getting braces is a big decision, so you should be well-informed.

This short book is from one parent to another. I have five children myself, and I know how important their health and happiness is. I think about it daily! This is a short but very informative guide on orthodontic treatment. I will explain the reasons one should get braces, what happens during the process, and how to cover the cost without breaking the bank.

I will do my best to educate you on the subject without using too much technical jargon. My goal is to answer any questions or concerns you may have about braces in this book.

The book itself has been broken up into four different sections. The first section is focused on helping you understand the benefits of orthodontics. In this section, we will cover many reasons for treatment, including common tooth and jaw problems that a lot of children experience.

The second section is a parent's guide to confidently navigating this big decision. You will learn some of the best ways to cover the investment of treatment.

The third section reviews the most common questions parents and patients have about the process of orthodontic treatment. We'll cover topics such as: how to take care of your teeth, how to keep your braces clean, and what to expect during the entire process, so that you walk away fully informed.

The last section covers what happens after orthodontics, and the process of keeping your teeth straight for the rest of your life.

I've written this book based off of years of working as an orthodontist, and thus dealing with the common questions I get from parents and patients. I base all of my commentary, treatment decisions, and recommendations off of the best and most current orthodontic research. My treatment recommendations are consistent with the American Association of Orthodontics, the American Board of Orthodontics, and the American Dental Association. I stay on top of the latest research and developments in the field of orthodontics so I can ensure you (or your child) gets the quickest and most enjoyable experience possible with orthodontic treatment. Let's go!

INTRODUCTION

We have a saying in our practice to "Serve PIE Daily!" This doesn't mean that everyone gets a piece of pie, although we do love pie in all of its varieties. What serving P.I.E. in our practice means is to have Positive Impact on Everyone! Our employees should have positive impact on each other, and on each our patients. Our patients should subsequently have positive impact on the community and their families. This is the purpose of our practice and why I chose to be an orthodontist. Orthodontics has tremendous benefits for those who receive treatment and will positively impact your life!

My first experience with the benefits of braces or Invisalign began in my senior year of high school. My younger sister, Dianne, was a freshman at the time. I did my best to be a great older brother to her. I would introduce her to friends, and protect her if she got picked on. I remember worrying about whether or not she felt accepted. Fitting in is emotionally consuming at that age! You see, my amazing sister had an upper front tooth that stuck out sideways. Unfortunately, even some of our own family affectionately called it her "snaggletooth" without realizing how self-conscious it was making her. It must have done a number on her confidence.

I remember the times being around her at school or out in town. She seemed so nervous and afraid when having interactions with anyone other than immediate family. It was painful for me to watch my smart, funny, and beautiful sister become a bumbling, fearful, emotional wreck with every new social situation.

It is unfortunate but true that an unattractive smile can be a social handicap. Appearance, especially facial appearance, can make a difference in the way people are treated or judged. People make this judgment within seconds. Often, it is subconscious and unintentional. This happens with everyone around us including students, teachers, co-workers, even total strangers, and ourselves. For example, people dress nicely, wear makeup, and comb their hair to improve the judgments people make about them. This is the biggest reason people get braces! It is one of the easiest ways to make a permanent positive change that will impact every social interaction for the rest of your life.

I treat a lot of children and teens in my office. When I talk to them, you'd be surprised how many of them are eager and excited to go through treatment. They recognize the benefit of a great smile, and many want braces to avoid future embarrassment. Because of the sensitive nature of being picked on, many children are just not willing to tell their parents about it. Most children have some nice friends and classmates. But it takes just one mean kid who picks on him/her about the way they look to really mess with their confidence. That's it! Just one mean, unkind, insecure bully. From that time forward, in the back of their mind, they always will remember the negative remarks. I can still think back to junior high and remember the comments made to me by cruel kids. For some reason, we don't hear and remember all the great things people say; it's just the pain that sticks with us.

John Gottman, a notable psychologist, did an analysis of married couples' likelihood of getting divorced or remaining married on a long-term basis. He found the single biggest determinant is the ratio of positive to negative comments the partners make to one another. And the optimal ratio is five positive comments for every negative one. For those who ended up divorced, the ratio was about three positive comments for every four negative ones. I would like to someday do a study on the interactions of kids at school. Happy children are probably getting a similar ratio to the couples that stay married, and unhappy children are dealing with a lot of negativity in their lives.

This research does not even take into account how individuals view and think about themselves. When you look into the mirror, what do you say? Do you say "I look great!" or "I hate the way I look?"

After high school, I went away on a two-year mission for my church. During that time, I didn't see my family. When I returned, I noticed something different about my sister. Dianne had become a more confident and outgoing person. She was much happier. I was shocked at the transformation in her personality, almost like a caterpillar becoming a butterfly. I couldn't figure it out at first, but after a week of being home, I asked my mother what had changed. She said, "Her snaggletooth is gone!"

That was it. The key to salvaging her self-esteem was straighter teeth! My parents, to their credit, recognized this was a problem for Dianne. Then they did something about it. Now everyone else knows

Dianne as I know her: a smart, funny, outgoing, and amazing person!

Seeing this dramatic change for my sister Dianne was awesome and life-changing for me as well! What an incredible blessing that orthodontist was for her at that time. In that moment, I decided that I wanted to have the same impact on people. I wanted to positively impact the lives of others.

Now, as an orthodontist, I get to see this transformation occur every day for many people. I love what I do. There is a tremendous amount of satisfaction to be gained by helping people increase their quality of life. Seeing the transformation that many kids make from the first time I meet them is still amazing to witness. From self-conscious and shy to vibrant and self-confident. It's a blessing to play a part in it all.

SECTION 1

Why People Get Orthodontics

DR. MATTHEW R. WIRIG

CHAPTER 1

*Why should I get braces for
my child or myself?*

Do you ever worry about your children? Do you ever wonder if you have done everything you can for them? Do you know what happens with them at school? Do they make friends easily, or do they sit alone at lunchtime? Do bullies pick on them? And why do they get picked on? Is it because they are shy or quiet? Is it because they have too much energy? Or is it the way they look? I have five children, and I can tell you my wife and I are kept awake at night worrying about these things. **Most of the time, we feel powerless to help!**

Secrets to be being a better parent

It was a dry, warm evening in May. My family was sitting around the dinner table when I noticed my daughter Brooklynn looking upset. I asked her what was wrong, and she let me know *she was being teased at school because of a crooked tooth*. Yes, you guessed it, just like my sister was 20 years ago. She was distraught about a front tooth that was slightly sideways. My daughter was nervous and hesitant to point it out to me because she was embarrassed, but my wife insisted she tell me.

How did I miss this? I am an orthodontist who straightens teeth every day. In my defense, I was always aware of that tooth, but I was putting it off until she was a little older. What I didn't expect was another kid would tease her at such a young age and embarrass her at school. She was only 9 years-old. The question I asked myself was, "Could I have prevented this humiliation?" I had all the tools and opportunity to prevent it, but my lack of action resulted in my daughter being humiliated and mocked at school, *and she didn't even feel comfortable telling me about it.* Obviously, I'm not the perfect parent! I want to give you the opportunity to prevent this from happening to your child too.

I'd like to start by clearing up some misconceptions about braces. Misconceptions about braces abound. Many people don't even realize that they could benefit from braces because it's not just about the looks. There are three main benefits to getting braces or Invisalign from an orthodontist.

Aesthetics

The first and most obvious reason for getting braces is to look better. This is the number one reason people get braces. It was the reason I put braces on my daughter Brooklynn, and the reason my sister Dianne got braces.

Could negative social experiences lead to lower self-esteem and a lower self-image? **The answer is yes!** And it's why people want straighter teeth. I realized by putting off the inevitable, I was actually bringing heartache and embarrassment to my daughter's life. Fair or not, it is true that appealing, good-looking people are generally perceived to be more intelligent, friendlier, more honest and trusting, and even more ethical. It's sad that society places so much value on appearance, but it's true.

People who smile more are happier. Many studies show that people who smile more are happier, do better in school and in college/university, and do well in job interviews too. The list of proven benefits is almost endless, and includes longer life, better health, and even more meaningful relationships. Great smiles are priceless and have a guaranteed return on the investment!

It's amazing that someone will buy an expensive outfit or designer clothes to make themselves more attractive or will spend thousands of dollars a year on hair care products, highlights, haircuts, and makeup, yet they may neglect improving their smile. A great smile is with you 24 hours a day, 7 days a week for an average of about 80 years. If you go through the process and wear retainers, you can keep that smile for as long as you live. I can't think of a better investment.

I don't want to understate the power of this advantage, but that is not the end of it. There are other reasons to get braces that deserve consideration as well.

Function

This is often overlooked by much of the general public. We use our teeth on a daily basis to feed ourselves. Chewing is an extremely important part of this process. It is impossible to go through a normal day without needing to utilize the functional part of our teeth and bite.

Teeth often need orthodontic treatment in order to work properly and efficiently. Crooked teeth and poor bites can lead to long-term, painful problems. These problems can include headaches, tooth and jaw pain, biting and chewing problems, and more.

The jawbone has a joint called the Temporomandibular Joint, known as the "TMJ." It is an extremely complex joint with the potential for many painful problems. These problems can be worse when teeth are not properly aligned. When the teeth are straight and the bite is corrected, it allows the joint to move more freely.

Health

Straight teeth are much easier to clean and maintain. This is great news. Orthodontic care is likely to save you money from dental visits, and the potential pain and cost associated with some tooth and gum issues throughout your life. It's much easier to minimize and prevent bone defects and health issues in the mouth later in life when you have straight teeth.

Crooked, crowded, and misaligned teeth are just harder to clean, brush, and floss properly. This can lead to even more serious problems than a cavity or two. It can also lead to gum loss. In extreme cases, it can lead to a buildup of harmful bacteria which increases your risk of complications from cardiovascular disease. Hard to believe, but true.

This doesn't leave you off the hook for maintaining the standards of proper oral hygiene (e.g. flossing and brushing regularly). It also doesn't mean you will never get another cavity if you get orthodontic treatment. It simply makes the time spent flossing and brushing easier and more effective. It also slows the buildup of plaque, helps gums to remain healthy, and decreases the chance of some tooth decay and bacterial growth.

Lastly, crooked or misaligned teeth can wear unevenly over the years, causing long-term problems with teeth. When the bite is not fitting, some teeth will be subject to excessive force, causing permanent damage and wear. Orthodontic treatment is an important part of long-term oral health.

So, as you can see, there are many benefits to having the perfect smile!

DR. MATTHEW R. WIRIG

CHAPTER 2

What are common problems corrected

by orthodontists?

Does your child feel like his or her teeth are crooked? Does your dentist say your child has a problem with his or her teeth which needs to be looked at by an orthodontist?

Like I mentioned in the previous chapter, there are misconceptions about receiving orthodontic care. Many people mistakenly believe braces are only for straightening crooked teeth. Along with straightening crooked teeth, orthodontists are able to correct any irregularities in the jaw and bite. Having these issues corrected early in life makes treatment easier on your child. Not to mention the long-term benefits of treatment like overall dental health and self-esteem.

I am constantly asked by parents, even friends and family, if certain dental conditions create the need for braces. The short answer is no. There are many problems that can occur with such a complex process. We have a set of 20 baby teeth developing and 32 permanent teeth replacing them. The teeth all need to erupt in the right order and location. At the same time, the jaw is growing and developing. Because it is so complex, it is extremely rare that everything goes perfectly. This all happens with the genes of two separate parents. I am amazed that more problems don't develop with such a complex process.

Braces or Invisalign may be suggested for your child, especially if he or she has any of the following conditions:

Crooked teeth

Teeth that come in crooked can embarrass your child, and they can cause problems down the road. In some cases, it's just one or two teeth that are crooked. Crooked teeth can be linked to various problems. They include difficulty eating and drinking, lack of self-esteem/confidence, increase in plaque buildup, and headaches. In extreme circumstances, health issues include back pain and heart problems.

Difficulty chewing food

Many common and easily corrected issues can cause difficulty with chewing food. This is not only inconvenient for eating, but it can lead to poor nutrition and other health problems. More complicated bite and jaw problems can make it hard to open and close your mouth.

Overbite or underbite

The upper teeth may extend beyond the lower teeth, causing the child to bite the roof of his or her mouth or cheeks. This is fairly common for children. It is estimated that 25-30% of children's orthodontic cases are linked to this uncomfortable issue. If this problem is severe enough, it may require surgery in conjunction with orthodontic treatment to fully fix the problem. If this is caught early enough by an orthodontist, surgery can often be avoided.

Crossbite

This is when the upper teeth sit inside the lower teeth and can cause misaligned jaw growth. When it happens in the back of the jaw, it is known as a posterior crossbite. In the front, it is known as an anterior crossbite. It can be one tooth or multiple teeth. As we chew, we put up to 200 pounds of pressure on our teeth. Failure to correct a crossbite can lead to painful problems in the future. A crossbite can also make the jaw growth uneven and make the face look crooked. Orthodontists will often recommend braces at an early age when faced with these problems for children. Solving this issue early on can eliminate a lot of problems and damage later on.

Do you bite the sides of your cheeks? How about your child? Doing so is a sign that the teeth are not properly aligned. This can be a very unpleasant problem to have. It can turn an otherwise enjoyable experience into a painful one quite suddenly.

Deep bite

A deep bite is when the upper teeth completely overlap and cover the lower teeth. This can be a severe problem if the lower teeth hit the roof of the mouth. When the lower teeth hit the roof of the mouth, it causes damage to gums on the roof of the mouth. This often makes eating and chewing very uncomfortable. Deep bites are often harder to treat than other types of bites, and may require longer treatment times.

Open bite

This happens when the front teeth do not touch, even when the back teeth are touching. This can cause difficulty with chewing, biting, and swallowing. Open bites can also cause speech problems.

If your child has an open bite, often you will notice his or her lips are not closed, even when the mouth is closed. Patients with open bites often comment on the difficulty of eating things as simple as a sandwich. They will not be able to cut through the lettuce or other things inside the sandwich, and the middle of the sandwich will pull out when they eat. This common condition is one of the more visibly noticeable ones, so it tends to lead to a lack of social confidence.

Spacing

Spacing is abnormal gaps in between the teeth (and in some cases, due to missing teeth). This is extremely common in young children, and it can actually be good to have some spacing while children are young. Because of this, spacing in teeth may not need to be addressed until the child is older. It is fairly straightforward to correct with braces or Invisalign. For more severe cases, it does help to treat the problem earlier and more aggressively. Treatment will be timed to allow for the best long-term results and management of the patient. There are many reasons spaces occur. Because of that, not all cases of spacing are treated the same. If your child has spacing, it is recommended to have your child's teeth and bite evaluated by an orthodontist.

My second oldest child, Carter, is almost ready to start braces because his two front teeth look like Mater's from Disney's animated movie, Cars. If you haven't seen the movie, Mater has a huge gap between his two front teeth. If the space between the two front teeth is 2mm or less, it will tend to be easier to fix. Unfortunately, his space is much larger and he will require braces to fix it. He is already begging me to get him in to fix it. He is only nine years-old, and he is becoming more aware of his appearance.

Crowding

Crowding happens when the teeth don't have enough room to fit within the jaw. They can struggle to emerge from the gum tissue and will not align properly on their own. At times, severe crowding will keep teeth from coming in. This is called a tooth impaction and can be very painful for a child. Crowding can make it difficult for your child to keep his or her teeth clean, and may aggravate any problems that are already present. Crowding is easily treated with orthodontics. In the vast majority of cases, tooth extraction can be avoided when the teeth don't have enough room to fit properly. In severe cases of tooth crowding, an eventual need for tooth extraction/removal may be required.

Premature loss of baby teeth

If your child lost his or her baby teeth early and the adult teeth did not come in for a while, this can lead to their new, adult teeth coming in crooked or poorly. This is something you should be on the lookout for just in case it happens to your child. Often, baby teeth are very useful at holding space for future permanent teeth. This is one of the main reasons we like to see kids, ages seven and above. If we catch problems like this occurring, we can make arrangements to hold the spaces with space maintainers. This will make things work out much better for a child during his or her treatment.

At times when a tooth is lost early, if the tooth on the opposite side isn't lost at, or nearly the same time, it can cause some shifting of the front teeth. We may have to extract another baby tooth to accommodate for the loss of a tooth on the opposite side.

Thumb sucking or pencil chewing

Thumb sucking can cause your child's front teeth to come in crooked. Pencil chewing is also not good for the teeth for the same reason. It's important to stop these habits as soon as possible, so that they don't create long-term problems. Chewing on things can also cause damage to your teeth.

At least once a week, a patient will come in, and I can tell within seconds that he or she still sucks his or her thumb. It's pretty obvious because the two front teeth will stick out quite far compared to the other teeth. Orthodontics alone will not fix this if the habit doesn't stop as well. It is important to stop thumb-sucking habits at around the age of four or earlier.

When I was 16, I was working at a movie theater. I was standing at a podium bored to death because all the movies had started and new ones wouldn't be starting for another hour. As I was standing there, I started foolishly chewing on a pen. In my boredom, I heard a crunch from my front two teeth. My heart stopped as I realized I had chipped a little piece of enamel from my front teeth. That was the last time I ever chewed on a pen or a pencil. So learn from my mistake and take my advice to avoid chewing on hard items.

Jaw shifts, clicking sounds, or the inability to open jaw

This can be a warning of a growth or developmental problem of the teeth or jaws, such as temporomandibular joint disorder (abbreviated as "TMD"). Orthodontists can examine and if necessary, treat it. Left unmanaged, TMD can be very uncomfortable or painful.

Injuries to the face

As your child's teeth are coming in, an injury to the face can cause them to come in crooked or incorrectly. If your child sustains an injury to the face, he or she should be taken to the dentist for an examination. The earlier any problems can be caught, the better. Recently, a friend of mine who had braces previously suffered a broken jaw in an accident. He will require braces again because of the damage to his jaw and bite. Injuries at times cannot be avoided. When they do occur, it's important to see if treatment is needed. If a tooth has been knocked out or moved significantly from an injury, then it is important for an orthodontist to begin moving it soon.

Genetics

Sometimes genetics play a role in the way your child's teeth develop. If you had problems with your teeth or needed braces, your child may as well. One of my favorite jokes that I hear frequently is when a mom brings a child into the office and tells me her child needs braces because the child got his or her father's teeth. It's funny because the fathers say the same thing about the mothers when the father brings in the child. The orthodontic profession exists because of parents with crooked teeth having children with crooked teeth. It's not your fault if you've had crooked teeth, and it isn't your child's fault either. Modern orthodontic treatment can correct the problems created by genetics. That's all that matters, and the way we treat our teeth is the only factor we can control.

Gum diseases

Gingivitis and periodontitis are rather serious dental problems. Periodontitis occurs when gingivitis is left untreated. Periodontitis (also known as "Periodontal Disease") is when the inner layer of the gums and bone pull away from the teeth and form pockets. These pockets can become infected and lead to a whole host of problems. If the teeth are not straightened early, your child is more likely to suffer from gingivitis and periodontal disease.

Many studies suggest a strong correlation between the buildup of certain types of bacteria in the mouth from gum-related diseases and heart disease. A person with periodontal disease is about twice as likely to have unsafe heart conditions including heart attack and stroke. The link is as strong as that of heart disease and cholesterol.

Other issues to be aware of

Having treatment to straighten the teeth and properly develop the jaw will help prevent other dental problems. For example, treatment can open the airways and prevent breathing problems. It also greatly reduces the risk of your child developing any of the following conditions: speech impediments, sleep apnea which is caused by mouth breathing and/or snoring, and grinding or clenching of the teeth, which can lead to tooth pain and/or loss.

If you or your child suffers from any of these conditions, you should make an appointment with an orthodontist to get an evaluation. The earlier any of these conditions can be diagnosed, often the easier and less expensive it will be for you to correct them. A person can get braces at any age, but many orthodontists prefer the process be done earlier while the teeth and bones are easier to move around. Younger patients tend to have quicker and easier treatments. Timing treatment initiation is very important; you don't want to start too late or too early.

Getting braces is no longer the painful or embarrassing event that adults may remember from childhood. There are many options available, and while there will be some discomfort, it does not have to be a painful experience. Getting braces does not have to hurt to mean it is working for your child. And with Invisalign, the comfort is even better.

We have technology that allows us to speed up the process of orthodontic treatment as well. Advances in technology, medicine, and science have made straightening teeth an easier and faster experience for patients.

CHAPTER 3

When is the best time to get braces?

The American Association of Orthodontists and the American Dental Association recommend that children have an evaluation by an orthodontist by the age of seven. Generally, the teeth and mouth haven't developed enough prior to that age to see many problems. Any later, and developmental problems may become really difficult to correct, and treatment will take longer than it needs to. However, each child is different, so these are just basic guidelines.

Most children will not need braces at age seven, but that's the age when we can start looking for potential problems that might be developing. Getting your child to an orthodontist at an early age is a great way to monitor his or her growth. We can take preventive measures that will minimize intensity, expense, and duration of future treatments.

For some, it may seem unnecessary to have your child seen this early. And honestly, for most kids, we do not need to begin any treatment that soon. But when we can catch something that no one else has seen, it can make a real difference. Orthodontists are trained to understand growth and development of the teeth and can visualize future results. I will often find problems that only need simple solutions at that age, and ultimately save time and money for families. I only recommend treatment for your children as if they were my own children.

If most kids don't receive treatment at age seven, the next question is, when will you recommend treatment, and when is the best time to get braces or Invisalign? Most orthodontists agree the ideal time for children to get braces is between the ages of 12 and 14. This is usually after your child has lost all of his or her baby teeth and the permanent teeth have had a chance to grow in. So basically, if we don't see any initial/early problems, we will want to wait to start braces when most or all of the permanent teeth have come in.

Why are so many kids getting braces at an early age?

I hear this question all the time from parents. While the number of people having braces is increasing with every generation, the number of kids at an early age is not necessarily increasing at the same rate. A few orthodontists believe in putting braces on all children at an early age. These orthodontists feel that every child should go through two phases of treatment, whether they have major problems at an early age or not. This is called multi-phase treatment. It is usually a two-step process. Phase one is normally at ages 7-10, and phase two is normally at ages 12-14.

The problem is that this form of treatment is based on old or unreliable data. It can cost more for families overall, and be more of a burden on children. Current research doesn't support the treatment of all children with multiple phases of treatment in this way. It is still a common practice among a few orthodontists though, so be sure to ask why a certain treatment is necessary at such a young age, and also if it is really needed twice. If you put braces on a child who still has baby teeth left, it lengthens the amount of time with braces on and can wear a child out from the treatment process, so that they are less compliant with treatment later on.

Personally, I don't recommend multi-phase treatments as a standard for all patients, as it can lengthen the overall time needed and increase the expense for parents. These recommendations are not just my personal opinions; they are supported by the American Association of Orthodontics and American Dental Association. If the orthodontic research supported phases of treatment, I would recommend it. But is does not, so we work hard to avoid unnecessary treatment. I mention it here because it is common enough among orthodontists that you could have some exposure to this type of philosophy.

However, there are times when orthodontics is really needed at an early age (7-10). This is why we recommend seeing children ages seven and above. A few problems, if not treated early, can lead to damage or an increase in problems later on. These problems include crossbites, impactions, irregular growth of the jaw, and other more rare occurrences.

If your child does need early treatment, the current orthodontic research suggests an "interceptive approach" which involves the use of dental appliances and/or some braces. This helps correct early problems while you wait for the baby teeth to fall out. Generally, we will only use the interceptive approach if your child's individual case is severe. Each case varies from person to person, so your young child most often won't even need the interceptive approach. If you are concerned at all, make sure to ask questions. Our goal is to make it as quick, painless, and convenient as possible for you and your child.

Is it too late for an adult to get braces?

There is no age limit for when a person can get braces. Many adults end up getting braces later in life, but the earlier you get them, the better. I have had a patient as old as 82. The truth is our bodies are easier to change the younger we are. This is because the bone is still developing and hasn't had the chance to completely finish growing up until our early adult years. This means that treatment in a child's teen years generally doesn't require as large an investment and is faster to complete. It is also less uncomfortable, the earlier it is started. If you get started when the teeth are ready, you have more years to enjoy the benefits of that great smile and the confidence that comes with it!

SECTION 2

What to Know Before You Get Treatment

DR. MATTHEW R. WIRIG

CHAPTER 4

*Should I get treatment from a Dentist
or an Orthodontist?*

It can be easy to confuse a dentist and an orthodontist. Orthodontics and dentistry are two separate professions. Almost every day, I have to explain what an orthodontist is, even to patients who are specifically trying to see one. Everyone knows what a general dentist does. A dentist fixes cavities and helps take care of your overall dental health. But unless you have had braces before, you may not know what services an orthodontist provides.

An orthodontist is a dental specialist. In fact, the American Dental Association and state boards recognize a number of different specialties in dentistry. The medical profession is the same as dentistry. A brain surgeon is a doctor, just as much of a doctor as a family doctor. But the brain surgeon specializes in fixing brains, while a family doctor handles more general illnesses and problems. A brain surgeon had to go to medical school just like the family doctor. But beyond the years spent at medical school, the two types of doctors have very different types of additional training.

If a person wishes to become an orthodontist, he or she must first become a dentist and complete dental school. Dental school is four years of education beyond a college/university bachelor's degree. After dental school, all graduates can practice as a dentist when they get licensed in their state. This is where the two professions become different. After becoming a dentist, an aspiring orthodontist must then complete an additional two to three years of specialized full-time study. This training in orthodontics is done in a residency program approved and accredited by the American Dental Association. It's very competitive to get into most residency programs, so it requires a dentist to score really high on exams and do very well in dental school to be admitted to an orthodontic residency. On average, there are 15 applicants for every single opening in an orthodontic residency program. In an orthodontic residency, an orthodontist learns how to correctly move a child's teeth and fix jaw-related problems using mostly non-surgical procedures. Orthodontics, and the study of straightening teeth, is always changing. Orthodontists are required by law to stay on top of any changes in our specialty and must complete a bunch of continuing education hours each year.

Once a residency is completed, an orthodontist is limited to only doing braces and Invisalign. So when I became a licensed orthodontist in the state of Nevada, I could no longer do general dental work, like fillings and cleanings. I received the same initial training as a dentist, but with the extensive training in orthodontics, orthodontists limit what they do to only moving/straightening teeth. Dentists are legally allowed to provide orthodontics too, but their experience is often very limited and they usually have little, if any formal training. In fact, most dentists refer their patients who need orthodontics to a licensed orthodontist for orthodontic treatment.

One question I get from a lot of people is "what do orthodontists actually do?" I get this question because dentists do most of the procedures on the patients. Patients can see the dentist doing the work. When you have a cavity filled, the dentist is the one drilling and filling the cavity. It can be confusing then to see an orthodontist who has his or her assistants perform most of the work on the patients. It's not uncommon in orthodontics to have 90% of the work done by the assistants. In orthodontics, it's not as important who is doing the work. What is more important is what is being done. Orthodontists are much more like architects who give the assistants the directions for the teeth to move safely and correctly. An orthodontist sets up a plan on how to correct the teeth and visualizes how the teeth will look in the end. It requires a completely different skill-set and training.

Only about 6% of general dentists become licensed orthodontists. As an orthodontist, I straighten teeth all day, every day. So I've become really good at what I do. In fact, many dentists and hygienists trust me to treat them and their own children.

Conversely, I send my wife and children to the dentist to get checkups and cavities filled. I trust dentists to take care of the overall dental health of my family. When it is time for braces, they will see me. My father-in-law still laments over the fact that I specialized to become an orthodontist. I think he was looking forward to free lifetime dental work when I started dental school, but now he has to go to someone else for his cleanings and dental work.

DR. MATTHEW R. WIRIG

CHAPTER 5

What happens at the initial appointment?

The following is an outline of what you can expect if you were to come in to my practice for a consultation.

The initial consultation generally takes one hour to complete and is free ($300 value). An hour may be difficult to find in your week, but it's an hour well invested in your child's oral health, social confidence, and happiness. The orthodontist will examine your child's mouth, their bite, and their facial and oral characteristics. This is done to see what procedures may need to be performed.

When you arrive to our office, one of our very friendly staff will greet you. We are expecting each and every new patient and plan our day around your appointments. Our goal is to make you and your child as comfortable as possible. It can be scary going to the orthodontist, but we're really nice people! So one of the first things we will do is give you an office tour so that you are comfortable with your surroundings. It's also a chance to ask questions about our doctors and other orthodontic related questions.

In the consultation, the orthodontist will require your child's dental records. As a parent, you will have to fill out a couple of short forms. Don't worry, we don't give you a mountain of complicated paperwork to fill out. This just gives us basic information such as your address, name, what insurance you carry, and other vital information. You are also giving the orthodontist permission to perform the necessary exams and procedures on your child. They cannot do this without your permission. The office may require your dental insurance card if you have one, so be sure to bring that with you.

During or before the consultation, X-rays of your child's mouth will be taken from different angles. This is a completely painless procedure and nothing for your child to be frightened about. The procedure only takes a few minutes, and now with digital x-ray technology, there is very little waiting time on the x-rays to develop.

We will also need the staff to take digital photographs of your child's teeth. This is done by inserting plastic cheek retractors into the patient's mouth to allow us to see the teeth. And then we photograph them. This is usually a simple and painless process.

The orthodontist then will examine your child's mouth and have the assistant record what he or she reports. This only takes a couple minutes. After the exam is complete, the orthodontist will speak with you and your child about what procedures may need to be done. Don't be afraid to ask questions. The orthodontist is there to help you and your child.

During the question and answer session, the orthodontist will discuss treatment options and plans for your child. This helps you create an individualized treatment plan that is unique to your child and created to yield the best possible results. At this time, the orthodontist will give you an estimated length of the treatment needed.

Remember, this is just an estimate. Sometimes this time can run over or under. It all depends on what treatment is needed, how the patient's body responds to treatment and how carefully you and your child follow the treatment plan and instructions.

The staff will next discuss financial information and insurance options to help cover the cost of the procedures. Orthodontists generally charge on the complexity of the procedures they have to perform so the more information and options you have available, the better it is for you. Most orthodontists accept payment plans, so do not be afraid to discuss payment options if you do not have insurance or insurance does not cover as much as you'd like them to. At our office, our goal is to make orthodontic treatment as convenient and affordable as possible.

As a convenience, some offices offer to start treatment the same day as the initial consultation. We do this because it saves you from having to come to a separate appointment. We block off time in the schedule to always allow someone to start the same day. We find parents like it because it saves time. We do this because I personally appreciate when my time is valued, and I'm sure you do too.

Time is something we value of yours. So, we make it a point to stay on our schedule as best as we can. We track waiting times in the office because it is so important to us and we are always looking for ways to be more efficient, along with providing great service and pleasant results!

DR. MATTHEW R. WIRIG

CHAPTER 6

What options are there for braces?

With today's modern orthodontics, there are many different options available for your child, including Invisalign, lingual braces, ceramic or clear braces, as well as traditional braces. In this chapter, I want to share with you all the options. Orthodontic treatments have come a long way from the older, clunky, and uncomfortable braces that our parents and grandparents had to wear. Braces today are smaller, more comfortable to wear, and are less likely to stain teeth. Let's take a look at some of the options available to you and your child.

Traditional metal braces

Traditional metal braces are now smaller and work better than they did in the past. They are still the most common type of treatment for straightening teeth and correcting bites. The metal brackets are attached to the teeth with an adhesive that binds them to the teeth. A wire runs across the brackets. The wire will be gently tightened to pull the teeth into their proper position. The metal bracket is simply an anchor site for the wire. If you have had braces, you probably remember the experience. Thanks to advances in modern orthodontic technology, braces are much less uncomfortable than in the past!

Depending on your age, you might remember the metal bands that went all the way around a person's teeth. Today, the metal bands only go around the four back teeth and are no longer used for the rest. Many patients never get any bands at all.

Metal brackets are made from a medically safe stainless steel. It is extremely rare to have any type of allergy develop because of the contents of the alloy. Often, if the patient does develop inflammation, it is caused from something other than the braces. If your child has a severe metal allergy, gold-plated or titanium braces are also available. These alternatives work exactly the same as their traditional counterparts but just cost more. In our office, the primary option for patients with allergies is ceramic braces, which we will discuss in the next section.

Modern metal braces also come with customizations. Patients can pick out the color of the bands that go around the bracket. Your child will have fun personalizing what colors he or she wants to use. Your child can even choose from a variety of colored elastic rubber bands. Some kids really have fun with this!

Metal braces are among the most affordable and quickest treatments available for your child. There may be some mild irritation within your child's mouth in the beginning. This irritation will go away very quickly as your child learns to live with the braces. In no time, your child may hardly even notice or feel the braces. I see many kids who are never bothered at all by the process. But most will be mildly annoyed, especially at the beginning. Adults, for the most part, get more annoyed by braces, and this is why Invisalign is so popular for adults.

Ceramic or clear braces

Ceramic, or clear braces, are made to blend in with your teeth. This makes them much less noticeable. If your child likes color, he or she can still customize them like metal braces with different colors. With ceramic or clear braces, the only thing that is really visible is the wire that runs across the brackets.

Ceramic or clear braces are made from ceramic or plastic alloys. They are similar to glass and tend to be more brittle than metal braces. Ceramic braces, unlike traditional braces, do not absorb force as well. Because of this, some orthodontists will avoid placing ceramic braces on your child's lower or back teeth where the child will bite down harder.

To account for the material properties of ceramic or clear braces, the brackets are often made a little thicker than their traditional metal counterparts. While this is not very noticeable to many patients, it is something for you to be aware of if you are considering clear or ceramic braces for your child.

Ceramic or clear braces also require more caution while eating, as the elastics that are changed at each appointment can stain. Stains appear due to foods like tomato-based soups/sauces, tea, coffee, red wines, curries, or anything else that stains. This will cause the small elastic ring around each brace to change color, usually yellowish. This happens with metal braces too, but is much less noticeable because the brace isn't clear. We change your elastics at each appointment, so you get a new, fresh, and clean set of elastics every time around the braces.

Lingual braces

Lingual braces are metal braces that attach to the back of the teeth instead of the front. They are often attached to the back of the teeth with gold or another metal alloy, and are not very visible from the front. A person would have to tilt his or her head backwards and let someone see the lingual (back or tongue) side of the teeth. These types of braces are not very common and are very expensive. It generally costs up to twice as much to have lingual braces as it does to have standard braces or Invisalign.

Lingual brackets have to be custom-made for each person's mouth using a mold the orthodontist makes. Because of the specialized, custom nature of lingual braces, they are more expensive.

Lingual braces are not suitable for patients who have a small mouth or certain tooth shapes. They can also interfere with the tongue's natural movements.

Not every orthodontist works with lingual braces. This is because few patients choose lingual braces, when you have other options like Invisalign. Invisalign is so much more comfortable and almost as invisible.

Six Month Smiles

Six Month Smiles is a trademarked brand name company that was created by a general dentist and is primarily marketed by general dentists. It is represented as an alternative to full orthodontic treatment offered by orthodontists. But it is really not the same thing at all.

To become a Six Month Smiles provider, a dentist must take a two-day paid course and then can market him or herself as a Six Month Smiles provider, unlike the two-to-three-year formal residency orthodontists take. This treatment, in reality, is a limited/minor treatment to correct minor issues with crowding. It can be somewhat confusing to some of the general public who don't know much about orthodontics.

Traditional braces straighten teeth and correct the bite of the patient. It is comprehensive. Six Month Smiles only slightly straightens some of the front teeth, and does nothing for the bite. Orthodontists can offer the same type of treatment for their patients, but we usually recommend full treatment instead. This is because of the benefits and long term stability of bite correction.

It's important to communicate your goals with the orthodontist. If you just want a few teeth straightened, then they can do that. I can't speak for all orthodontists, but I have found that when comparing Six Month Smiles with the same type of limited treatment in my office, I can often do it for less cost, in shorter time, and with the best results possible. So it is important to compare apples to apples, and inquire if the provider is a dentist or an orthodontist, and to know what results will be achieved when looking into Six Month Smiles.

DR. MATTHEW R. WIRIG

CHAPTER 7

Everything you need to know about Invisalign

Invisalign has been all over the news lately. Everyone has been hearing about its benefits. Invisalign can be used to treat crossbites, overcrowding, overbites, underbites, openbites, and gaps in the teeth. I've reserved an entire chapter to talk about it because it is such a great product. There's a lot to cover, so let's get started.

Invisalign is different from traditional braces. The orthodontist will use a computer to create a 3D digital model of the teeth and bite. The model will be used to simulate how the teeth will be moved into their final position.

Invisalign is a set of plastic mouthpieces called "aligners" that gently push the teeth into place. The aligners may be referred to as trays, or even just mouthpieces. Typically, a person will need a series of 10 to 50 sets of these aligners to correct his or her teeth. With a 3D computer model and the simulation, Invisalign trays will be custom-made for each patient. The patient gets a new aligner every two or so weeks as prescribed by the orthodontist. These trays are practically invisible, hence the name Invisalign.

In order to use Invisalign, there are two ways to capture the shape and position of your teeth to create, plan and start your treatment. The first way is to take a mold or impression of your teeth, and the second way is to take a computer-aided 3D scan of your teeth.

The older method is an impression or mold of the teeth. This means we would take a mold and fill it with some gooey plastic-like material that becomes solid after a few minutes. The gooey material is placed in the mouth of the patient and pressed onto the teeth. The material stays over the teeth for a few minutes, then the dental assistant will wiggle it off, pulling the tray away from the teeth and out of the mouth. It can be kind of awkward and uncomfortable sometimes. On top of that, the patient has a bunch of gooey stuff left over to clean up on the inside of the mouth and lips.

This creates a detailed type of impression. It can be an effective technique, but it can also be sensitive and uncomfortable for patients. Due to the nature of the impression material and method, there is sometimes a need to take additional impressions if an impression doesn't come out just perfect. That can mean longer and/or additional appointments. Because of the limitations on comfort and accuracy of traditional impressions, our practice uses a better way.

So let's discuss the newer 3D scanning method. I'm obsessed with making everything in our office as quick and convenient as possible for our patients. So we decided to move on to a better impression system once it became available. In 2013, Invisalign started integrating with iTero. iTero is a digital scanner that takes multiple 3D images of the teeth. It is a lot more comfortable than the old way. No gooey liquids or molds are involved. It is also a lot more accurate, meaning fewer problems and faster, better results.

Most practices don't invest in the iTero scanner because it can be very expensive, although more switch over all the time. I saw this as a must-have because my patients deserve the best! If it's better for the patients, it's better for us too. The turnaround time for Invisalign is much faster now as well because we don't have to ship impressions back and forth to the Invisalign offices.

When you start treatment, the Invisalign trays must be worn an average of 22 hours a day. They should only be removed for eating, drinking, and brushing teeth. The only exception is drinking water, which you can do with the trays in.

Another feature of Invisalign is the attachments we bond or glue to your teeth. Attachments are little tooth-colored bumps of hard material. They come in all shapes and sizes, and are generally very difficult to see. These attachments work with the trays to apply pressure on the teeth.

There are many advantages to Invisalign over traditional braces.

The first advantage is they are a lot more comfortable for most people. Irritation of the gum tissue and cheeks is low with the aligners/trays. Additionally, the overall soreness has been shown to be significantly less. You may experience some soreness with each new set, but the discomfort goes away quickly and is less intense.

Another advantage is the ability to clean your teeth without having to navigate around braces. Patients being treated with Invisalign simply remove the aligner/tray. From there, they can floss and brush as anyone without braces would. This is a much faster process than cleaning around braces.

You don't have the same eating restrictions with Invisalign. There are no brackets or wires to break. You eat without your trays in. Traditional braces can have a tendency to get food stuck in and around them as well. You don't experience this with Invisalign.

Invisalign gives patients more flexibility with playing certain musical wind instruments, snorkeling/scuba diving, and with certain sports that require special mouthpieces.

However, the biggest advantage is the reason everyone wants to get Invisalign. They are clear and practically invisible! This feature is highly sought after by patients. It appeals to adults and teens alike.

Few people will ever know you are wearing them. This makes them very popular for brides to be who are planning for an upcoming wedding. In the past, we might put braces on a woman who is engaged, take them off for the wedding, and put them back on afterwards. All this to accommodate the pictures and experience of her special day. Now, brides can wear their Invisalign trays throughout the day of their wedding and nobody is the wiser.

I've dealt with similar situations for those with quinceaneras, proms, senior pictures, and other special events occurring in their near future.

Professionals, models, and TV personalities love Invisalign too. They can maintain their image and improve their smiles without even having to remove their trays. There isn't a day that goes by when I'm watching TV that I don't see someone wearing Invisalign. Pretty much the only person trained to spot someone wearing Invisalign is an orthodontist who does a lot of it. But then again, I notice a lot more about people's teeth than the general public. If we meet in public, don't be bugged if I can't stop staring at your teeth, I am always diagnosing and evaluating everyone's smile around me.

Invisalign can cost slightly more than traditional braces, but they generally also require fewer appointments with your orthodontist. Treatment times vary for different people and depends a lot on the objectives the patient wants to achieve. Generally, Invisalign and traditional braces take the same time to complete treatment. The factor that limits how fast we can move teeth is each person's individual body and metabolism.

My personal preference is for patients to choose Invisalign when it comes to straightening teeth. I've been through treatment with it and it was a great experience for me. I recommend it to anyone wanting to straighten his or her teeth.

Moms are getting Invisalign

We are seeing a lot of moms getting Invisalign lately as well. Especially once they are done having children. You may or may not know this, but a woman's teeth often shift during pregnancy. This can create new problems for a woman, even if she has had braces in the past.

I've even been asked to speak formally to mothers and "mommy bloggers" on this subject by Invisalign.

My wife started treatment with Invisalign after she gave birth to our fifth child. She'd had braces when she was younger. Here are some of her thoughts on her Invisalign journey:

"I wore a retainer faithfully for years until I had my first child. The morning sickness was so bad for me that I remember thinking there was no way I could put that old retainer in my mouth. So, like many others who had previously had braces, I stopped wearing my retainer. Eleven years and five children later, my teeth had moved. A lot!

When I spoke to my husband about getting braces, he suggested Invisalign. I was very excited about it since I remembered all too well the frustrations I had with traditional braces. It's been a great experience! I saw an improvement in my teeth in as short as a couple months' time. It took me a short time to learn how to speak correctly with the aligners in, but that was no longer an issue in a matter of days.

My favorite thing is being able to take them out in order to eat. I also like that they are clear because nobody notices them. Having had braces in the past, I am amazed at how easy it has been with Invisalign. I would definitely recommend Invisalign to anyone who is wanting to get their teeth straightened. It's an easy process to go through and I am super happy with my results. I really haven't had any noticeable discomfort, I couldn't be happier."

Wirig Orthodontics is a premier provider for Invisalign. It's a product I believe in and strongly endorse because of the convenience and advantages offered.

Invisalign Teen

You may have heard about a new type of treatment by Invisalign called "Invisalign Teen." It is quickly becoming the cool thing for teenagers to have instead of traditional braces. The positive buzz about it has been great. I definitely think teens are pushing for it with their parents. It wasn't long ago that only parents had cell phones. Now, every kid from junior high school and up has one too.

This is the same thing that is happening with Invisalign, and Invisalign Teen. Invisalign Teen is a relatively new product from Invisalign. The technology is the exact same product as traditional Invisalign. The only difference is that it has some additional features that make it more applicable for teenagers. The Invisalign Teen treatment option gives the doctor more flexibility with baby teeth falling out and permanent teeth coming in, so it can be helpful for treatment when a patient has a couple of baby teeth left.

Invisalign Teen also has what are called "compliance indicators." Compliance indicators are little blue dots in the Invisalign trays that tell the doctor if the trays are being worn an effective amount, in general. The blue dot is a special compound that disappears over time from contact with a patient's saliva. They turn from blue to clear. This helps us keep the teens accountable to wearing the trays enough hours each day.

The other main difference with standard Invisalign is the Invisalign Teen product also includes up to five replacement aligners. This is in case the trays are lost or damaged. Invisalign added this feature to gives moms peace of mind so they can avoid the cost of replacement aligners. Invisalign published a case study that showed that moms were concerned with the reliability of teens. So Invisalign added these features for that reason. Of all the teens we have treated, the included replacement aligners have proven to be more than enough, saving parents from having to cover the cost of more replacement aligners. Invisalign Teen has been an overwhelming positive experience for our patients.

The wonderful thing about Invisalign lately is the overall low amount of pain it causes. It really is awesome!

CHAPTER 8

How do you cover the cost of braces?

Wondering how you will pay for braces can be stressful. There are many convenient ways for you to cover the cost of braces and not break the bank.

Orthodontic insurance can be really helpful with the costs of treatment. We accept pretty much every orthodontic insurance available. We do this because we want to eliminate as many barriers as possible for parents and families. With hundreds of insurance carriers and types of plans, it is impossible to explain every scenario in this book. Not all dental insurance covers orthodontics, but when it does, generally, the insurance will cover 25% up to 50% of the treatment costs, while you will pay the remaining portion out of pocket. Some orthodontists offer payment plans for the patients' portions (we do), and will bill your insurance for you by filing all the necessary claims (we do that as well). Don't be afraid to ask about all of your options.

That being said, lower cost does not always mean better value or even the same treatment. Be sure you find an orthodontist who has a good reputation. Good online reviews are one place to start. Talking to friends, neighbors, and other dentists is also a good way to get a recommendation. A good orthodontist will have nothing to hide and can often provide you with references if you ask for them.

Insurance

There are so many variables to insurance and costs. Every insurance policy has specific rules for different things. Some require waiting periods for benefits to kick in, like making you wait a year before you can get braces. Some require preauthorization from the insurance office to allow for the insurance to pay. Some have age limits on when you can get braces. Some even require you to see your dentist at least twice before being referred to the orthodontist.

Insurance companies have developed strategies to pay out less in benefits overall. Their aim is to increase profits for shareholders. The more rules they have, the more complicated it is; thus, the less people will use it. If you do not play the game by the rules they set up, then they will not pay.

It's important to know the rules for your specific plan. Some orthodontists do not take insurance because it's such a hassle. And for many, if they do take insurance, they only take the really easy ones rather than more difficult ones. I have to employ multiple full-time staff members just to handle insurance for patients. As a business owner, it is a huge cost, but I think the benefit for my patients is tremendous; it allows so many people a more affordable solution to having orthodontic treatment.

If you have dental insurance, many programs will cover part of the cost of your child's orthodontic treatments. Some plans will cover up to $3,000 of treatment, but most average around $1,500. If you are uncertain, you should look up your insurance policy to see what and how much is covered. You may need to speak with a customer service representative or you can have our staff do it for you. Some offices like ours file your insurance claims for you, making the complex process of using your insurance more manageable. Not all offices do this, so it is important to ask beforehand. Our staff is really good at figuring out insurance; it's what they do all day – calling to verify benefits and understand the rules of each one.

Secondary Insurance

Many patients may be covered under two dental insurance plans with orthodontic benefits. This happens for children with two parents or responsible parties who have two separate insurance plans. One policy is designated and viewed as the primary policy, while the other policy is the secondary policy.

The determination of which policy is the primary policy is based on which parent has the earliest birthday in that year. If my wife and I both had separate dental insurance policies, hers would be the primary because her birthday is in February and mine would be the secondary because my birthday is in December. This is a universal insurance rule that cannot be modified. The claim is submitted to the primary insurance first to determine the amount of benefit that the primary insurance will pay. Once an EOB (explanation of benefits) is mailed to the parent and the orthodontist, a new second claim is then submitted to the secondary insurance with the EOB from the primary insurance. The new claim will be adjusted based on the amount paid by the primary insurance.

The orthodontic benefit paid from the secondary insurance varies greatly under each insurance carrier's rules. While some secondary insurance carriers will pay the full orthodontic benefit, others will pay a percentage to none of the benefit due to the primary insurance payment.

Responsible Parties

When you begin treatment, you will be required to sign a contract for any treatment fees and an explanation of office policies. Most contracts have one responsible party who will pay the balance of the treatment costs that are not covered by insurance. Some patients have up to two responsible parties splitting the total treatment costs. This is most common with divorced parents or when grandparents are assisting with costs. Sometimes offices will set up two accounts, but will require both parties to sign the financial contract in the full amount as a contingency. The main reason is that if one party fails to pay their portion, the responsibility of payment will be on the other responsible party. Other offices require one parent to be the responsible party alone and he or she would need to figure out the splitting of fees between the other party without involving the doctor, office, or staff.

Prepayment in Full

If you are interested, you can discuss a paid-in-full option with your orthodontist. Many orthodontic practices like ours offer a discount for paying upfront. It's a percentage off the total cost if you can pay in full or with cash. The cost of treatment will vary depending on the complexity of your child's needs. If you want to pay everything all at once, you will also avoid interest charges, if any, on payment plan options. Not all orthodontists accept full payment up front, so make sure you ask about this option during the consultation phase.

Payment Plans

At our office, we offer plans that allow you to cover braces in monthly installments. We are willing to work with you on making sure that price isn't preventing you or your child from the smile you both deserve. Most of our payment plans have 0% interest and can be as low as $0 down.

Generally, our patients choose a plan that has them pay $500 as a down payment, and then they will divide the remaining balance (minus insurance benefit) by a certain number of months. The number of months usually correlates with how long the treatment is estimated to take. The more months, the lower the payments will be, and if the payments are larger, the faster the balance will be paid off. We offer auto-debit of checking accounts/credit cards to make it much easier to pay each month.

Extended Prepayment Plans

An option that is not very common, but that we are finding more helpful for families is to offer payment plans before treatment has begun. An example of how this works is when a parent brings a child in for an exam at age seven, and he or she is not ready for braces, but will need them in the future. Or when someone won't need braces for another year and he or she wants to get ahead of the costs by paying lower payments than he or she would normally have. In these types of cases, we can set up a payment plan for parents to put money toward braces long before they need them. We give parents a general idea of future costs and they can choose a monthly amount to be put towards braces in the future.

This type of creative payment structure would mean a payment amount less than usual each month, making it much more manageable, long-term. Most offices do not do this, but we do it because it has been really helpful for some families. If those families were ever to move or not need to use the payment towards braces, we refund the amount already saved up. We just want to give our patients another tool to make braces affordable for everyone.

Flex Spending Account

A flexible spending account is a popular benefit option offered by some employers. This is an account that allows participants to avoid taxation on money spent for procedures like braces. At the time of hiring at your employment, or during the annual open enrollment period, employees may elect to set aside a portion of their pay for a given year into a flexible spending account. It is important to plan ahead and know the amount you want to set aside. Whatever money is allotted into this account is free from all taxes. This means you cans save a significant amount on treatment.

The key to these accounts is to set it up with your employer before you begin treatment. It may take a little while to get things in place because some employers only enroll employees once a year, and if you missed it this year, you will have to wait until next year. The only way to change things midyear is if you have a major change in your family situation (i.e. divorce, birth, marriage, or other insurance coverage loss).

Then, once you have a plan in place, make sure you or your child is seen for an exam. That way, you know the costs of treatment (including other healthcare costs/needs) before you allocate money to the account. Remember, if you put too much in the account and end up not needing it, you lose it.

Third Party Financing

Another way to pay for braces or Invisalign is through third party financing companies. These companies specialize in issuing credit for orthodontics and other dental expenses. Some plans offer no down payments and extended payment plans. With extended payment plans, the monthly costs can be made really low.

This is primarily for patients who cannot afford the in-house payment plan's monthly payments. These companies have many attractive plans offering no down payments and extended payment plans. These companies typically issue a revolving line of credit for individuals and families. The amount of credit is based upon the patient's or responsible party's credit score. Some companies that issue these products include Chase Health Advance, Care Credit, Capital One Healthcare Finance, and Springstone Finance. Patients or orthodontic offices can submit an application to one of these companies and can be approved or declined in seconds. This is the preapproval process.

The advantage of using this method of payment is the ability to pay for orthodontic care without an initial payment or with really low monthly payments. Payment plans vary in terms of interest rate and length of repayment. There are even plans that have no interest for payment plans up to 18 months. The companies will charge your orthodontist a large fee to make up for the 0% interest for the shorter length plans. Some companies charge interest (2-28%) for payment plans that range from 24 months to 84 months. While extending monthly payments beyond the treatment time may provide patients with the ability to pay for treatment at low monthly rates, patients must understand that this comes with additional overall costs. Because of the costs of the fees to the practice and our patients, our offices try to make the in-house financing a better alternative.

"Medically Necessary" Orthodontic Coverage

With the Affordable Care Act, all children under the age of 19 are required to have basic dental care as a part of their health insurance policy. Medically necessary orthodontics is one of the 10 Essential Health Benefits (EHB) of all dental insurances. What this means is, if the child under the age of 19 has a case that is really serious, he or she may qualify for orthodontic coverage even if it's not a defined benefit of the insurance policy. So, the insurance would be required to cover the cost of braces.

To qualify as "medically necessary," scoring systems have been set up to for certain conditions.

Basically, if you get enough points as measured by the orthodontist and the insurance, then you could qualify. Only about 1 in 6 children would have severe enough need to qualify under this clause. If so, the orthodontist is required to submit a significant amount of information to the insurance. The insurance companies definitely don't make it easy. The orthodontist needs to complete a full write-up of the case and submit a lot of support materials to prove the child's need. This requires hours of work by the orthodontist without any guarantee of approval. The insurance company then takes the write-up and records submitted, and will either agree or disagree. If they disagree, then the child will not be deemed "medically necessary" and the claim will be denied. If they agree, then the insurance company will cover the necessary treatment costs.

Most orthodontic offices don't understand the benefit this could be to their patients, and therefore do not educate them on this possibility. Additionally because of the work involved, they may avoid submitting cases. You should inquire to see if your orthodontist is willing to participate should a child qualify for medically necessary treatment. In our practice, we always strive to do whatever we can to make orthodontics accessible to as many people as possible.

Other Options to get braces

Some government programs such as Medicaid will help cover the cost of orthodontics. Not all government programs make this easy, so be prepared to fill out a great deal of paperwork. If you have

Medicaid or another government program, it is best to get the authorization process started right away to reduce waiting time on what will and what won't be covered. Most orthodontic offices do not accept Medicaid because the amount the insurance reimburses for orthodontics is not enough to cover the expenses.

For low-income families, there is a program called "Smiles Change Lives." It's available in all 50 states. There are several important factors taken into consideration before you are accepted into the program. If approved, you will pay $600 for the administrative fees, and they will connect you with an orthodontist who provides his or her services and the orthodontic treatment for free. The child is introduced to the orthodontist by having an initial exam. The reason we do this in our practice is we feel it is important that we give back to the community. It's a great feeling to help those in need, when we can.

To qualify for Smiles Change Lives, you must meet the following criteria and apply:

- Your child must be between the ages of 11 and 18.

- A family of four must have an income of $40,000 or less or $10,000 per person.

- Parent(s) or guardian(s) must be willing to pay the $30 application fee.

- The child's teeth must be moderately to severely crooked.

- The child must take very good care of their teeth.

- The child must not have more than four baby teeth.

- The child must have no unfilled cavities.

Smiles Changes Lives providers only allow patients to use the traditional metal braces. A child will not be able to get Invisalign or any other type of special braces through this program.

DR. MATTHEW R. WIRIG

CHAPTER 9

What do you look for when picking an office

One of the main disadvantages for dentists or orthodontists as a whole is they have a habit of building the business around themselves and what is important to them. They may not work on Fridays or Saturdays because they enjoy their free time off. They may want to be done with work at 5pm like everyone else. I often cringe when I see a colleague who refuses to open the office occasionally on Fridays or Saturdays. Some practices don't want to pay credit card fees, so they may only accept cash, or they may not want to deal with insurance companies, so they will not accept insurance. It's just easier to have the world revolve around us.

That doesn't sit right with me. What we've built our practice around is three main key areas. These areas help my team and I focus on what is important for our patients. They are Convenience, Value, and Trust. When we make any business decision, we look back to these three keys. We want to build the practice around our patients instead of ourselves.

So we ask ourselves these important questions:

1. Does it make it more convenient for our patients?
2. Does it provide more value for our patients?
3. Does it create more trust for our patients?

If it doesn't hit the mark on one or more of those questions, we toss it out.

For example, one day a while back, I was discussing with my team if we should start to offer appointments on Saturdays. The question was answered when we related it back to our three keys. It definitely makes it more convenient and adds value as well.

Allow me to detail what we have done in these areas to create more convenience, value, and trust.

Convenience

We want to make it as easy as possible to do business with us. With this in mind, we wanted to eliminate all the barriers that normally get in the way. We offer appointments as early as 7am and stay open until 7pm at night. We offer appointments Monday through Saturday. This is important because many of our patients are in school or have jobs and work, and cannot miss time during normal business hours. We work hard to make it more convenient to get an appointment. The way we provide this is by having our staff and doctors rotate working at different times and on days like Saturday. Our staff pitches in to make it work better for you. It also makes Wirig Orthodontics unique from most offices out there.

Value

At our practice, we accept as many insurance and payment options as we possibly can. Our staff do a complimentary benefits check and submit all insurance claims for our patients. We accept every major credit card, and even things like CareCredit and

Springstone Financial. We offer in-house payment plans that are mostly 0% interest. It's cheaper to finance through us than it is to get financing on a car, or anything else for that matter. The only thing we ask for when we provide 0% interest is that you let us do auto-debit on a checking account or credit card. We do this for all of our patients, which means you never have to worry about paying your bill; we take care of it for you. This eliminates a lot of the billing hassles that can come up and saves our practice and you money. We even structure our payment plans to be as low as $0 down and can make your monthly payments fit your budget. Our treatment coordinators strive hard to make it convenient and affordable for you.

When you are done with your braces or Invisalign, we want you to be so excited to share your smile with everyone around you. It is important that you receive not only a great result but a great experience with as little pain, discomfort, and trouble as possible.

We have evaluated each of the areas of our practice and want you to receive a ton of value. An example of this is that we include two sets of retainers after treatment, for all patients. I felt horrible to learn about a patient of ours who had lost her retainer. Her teeth had shifted because she couldn't come see us for a few days due to finals.

Most orthodontists provide the minimum single set of retainers for their patients. I had done this for a couple years as well. My frustration and sympathy for that patient was why I made the bold decision that all of our patients will get two sets when they get their braces off. This has been one of the best things we have done as a practice. Rarely do we have patients who come in with shifted teeth. In fact, we started offering retainer insurance to help patients with the costs of lost retainers, and we have advised all patients to always have a backup retainer on hand in their homes.

We strive to make orthodontics an affordable situation and provide great results, but we also offer a clean, high-tech office. Our office is constantly being improved, and we regularly add new features to our facilities and services. We want the experience to be fun and inviting when you come to the office, as well as comfortable and friendly. This is why, in our offices, you will find iPads for kids and other cool things like a slushy machine. In fact, the future vision I have for improvements in the practice will see some huge changes to the offices. We are going to be moving to a more fun environment with the addition of lots of games and things for the patients and kids. If we could become an amusement park, we would.

We're always in the process of coming up with even more ways to provide value and make the experience more enjoyable as well.

Trust

It is important that you feel like your doctor and the team around them are the best that they can be. We invest heavily in the training of our staff and team. I've even had many staff members tell me that I have spent more money on their education than their own parents.

It is important that they provide the best customer service possible. I place a lot of importance on our doctors being trained beyond that of the average doctor. I do not believe in being mediocre or doing the bare minimum. As of this writing, all the doctors who work for our practice also teach at the post-graduate level. This means educational institutions trust us to teach orthodontics to other doctors. We believe in and are so passionate about this profession that we spend time teaching it. Our patients receive the best care available because of this.

DR. MATTHEW R. WIRIG

CHAPTER 10

"Dr. Wirig, if you were to be treated, what decisions would you make?"

This is really an interesting question. Growing up, I knew very little about braces or orthodontics. I grew up in a middle-class home, and there were so many of us, we were lucky to go to the dentist, let alone get braces. My mom worked full-time as a registered nurse, and my dad worked for the FBI as a special agent. I was the second oldest of seven kids, and I'm sure my parents just avoided the thought of getting braces because they didn't want to have to pay for all seven of us to get them.

Fortunately, the first couple of us, including myself, had relatively straight top teeth. The first three of us were boys, so maybe it didn't bug us that much that the rest of our teeth were really crooked. I can't remember even thinking about the process in high school, except once, when a friend of mine told me he was excited to get his braces off. I am amazed now I made it so far without thinking about braces. Of course, I was one of the lucky ones.

Since I have become an orthodontist, I have constantly been putting off getting braces. That was until the fall of 2013. I first decided I wanted to get it done because of some incredible enhancements and improvements in the process. As an orthodontist, I felt we finally had the perfect combination of treatments.

What is that combination? Allow me first to tell you about the things most important to me when it comes to my own treatment.

Comfort

I am a baby, and even as an orthodontist, I avoid going to the doctor whenever possible. Doctors and dentists often inflict pain (with the greatest of intentions!) on others and then send them home. They rarely have to see a great deal of the pain they inflict. I'm grateful that my patients tend to be braver than I am.

My older brother is a dentist. He is MY dentist, and even though he is in a different state, he is the one I see for my dental appointments. He can tell you I always complain to him constantly about pulling too hard on my cheek or not being able to get me numb. And because he is my brother, I am more honest with him about pain than I might otherwise be. Frankly, I think he is very good at what he does.

I've been on both sides of the chair, as a doctor and patient. So I take very good care to make treatment comfortable and enjoyable. I know what it's like to have painful prodding and poking going on in my mouth, and I don't like it. So, I'm very conscious of not delivering unnecessary pain to my patients.

Discretion

Part of my job is talking to hundreds of patients and parents a week. I also teach at the University of Nevada, Las Vegas in the orthodontic program, and I consult with other dentists on a daily basis. It is important to me that I don't feel self-conscious about my smile when talking to patients, parents, or other doctors. If you rated my vanity on a scale of 1-10, I wouldn't be a 10, but I also wouldn't be a 1. I don't want something to distract my patients from the message I am giving. And I definitely don't want patients, parents, dentists, or other orthodontists making fun of my smile either. See? Even being an adult now, I'm still aware of how my smile affects the perceptions of others. Imagine if my teeth weren't straightened; what would my patients think about that? I had felt trapped for a long time. I didn't want to have the slightest of crooked teeth, but I also didn't want to wear braces for the time it would take to fix them.

So what was the answer to the first two important factors for me? Well, it was to do Invisalign instead of doing traditional or clear braces. Invisalign is just far more comfortable and almost entirely discreet.

This is fairly common with adults. Braces are often seen as something that only kids get. This is why Invisalign is so popular with them, and it's because of Invisalign, I chose to straighten my teeth.

Time

I hardly ever get sick, it seems. However, if I did, I wouldn't see a doctor unless I absolutely had to. I hate sitting in waiting rooms. Maybe I am just impatient, but it drives me nuts. That's why you won't have to wait long in my waiting rooms. It is a huge focus of ours. One where you don't wait for hours because the doctor got behind. Although we are not perfect, I guarantee you will see a difference at our office when you compare it to most other medical experiences.

Let me share a quick story with you about my wife and our youngest child, Ethan who was born in January, 2014. Ethan had some problems when he was born and he was in the neonatal intensive care for a week until his breathing improved.

We have five kids, and this was the first time we've had a child who had to stay in the hospital with problems. There were times when we were a scared that he might not survive. He just struggled really badly at first and for the first couple days. As you could imagine, this was a stressful situation for my wife and I. When we were ready to leave, the doctors instructed us to have him checked by with the pediatrician the next week. One week later, my wife took our son to the pediatrician. Suddenly, I'm at my office when I get an unexpected call from my wife. She's just beside herself. She was crying in a way that she only does when she is very upset by something. It was a cry I rarely hear, and I knew something was very wrong in her world.

My wife showed up a little early to the pediatrician's office just to be sure she wouldn't be late and miss our son's appointment. When she got there, the waiting area was full of sick children. They were sneezing, coughing, wheezing, etc. Some of these kids were going to and from the restroom, throwing up, and sniffling. And our precious newborn who had just gotten out of the NICU had to stay in this environment! It was very unsettling for my wife.

I don't blame the other parents for taking their children to the doctor; that's what they should do and it's what I would do too. But this pediatrician was so backed up that my wife was forced to wait for hours to see him. And then, when she finally did get to him, he only gave Ethan a quick glance and sent my wife on her way.

My wife is an amazing woman. Hearing her on the phone, in tears, just broke my heart. She felt disrespected and hurt by this terrible experience. Our fragile newborn son needed added protection from sickness, not an increase in exposure.

At the time, when I was talking to my wife, I had people in my waiting room. They were waiting on me. I vowed to never put my patients in a situation like what my wife went through. We aim to have a really short waiting room times. We track the number of appointments that don't start on time and how many minutes late they start. We look at it every day. My team actually has to track the number every day in a report that I look over. If there's ever a problem, we track down what the problem was and fix it so that it doesn't happen again. My patients deserve the best, so my goal is to treat them the best with short waiting times.

Why don't most healthcare offices care about convenience, or respect other people's time? Recently, we polled our patients and asked what it was that kept them from getting braces or Invisalign sooner. You see those who do get treated are very grateful and excited to have straighter teeth. No one is upset about looking better. The thing that holds most of us back is life. Life gets so busy with school, work, and other activities.

How many times have you said to yourself, "There's just not enough hours in a day?"

We are just too busy to have our time wasted!

I get it. It's hard to imagine it being convenient to get braces for your child. It is a stress-filled, busy, hectic, tough, tiring, demanding, mind-numbing, energy-sapping battle each and every day out there, isn't it? I know – after all, I am a father and husband too.

The other aspect of time I was concerned about was overall treatment time. About two years is the general answer for patients when they ask how long it takes to straighten their teeth. I like to overestimate. Really, the average is less than that, but who wants to be in braces or Invisalign for anywhere near that long? In two years, the world is a drastically different place.

Whatever treatment I decided on, it needed to be fast. As fast as humanly possible! I was so excited about some of the new advances taking place because speed is important to me.

I've added two advanced treatments as options for patients like me: Acceledent and Propel. Both are aimed at stimulating the bone so that the teeth move faster. Both have documented research which shows they increase the speed of treatment by as much as half, for each. And because they are not the same types of treatment, I wanted to see how fast we could move teeth when they were all used together. More about that later in the book.

Comfort, time, discreet treatment, and aesthetics are the most important things to me. All of these things are very personal. I don't want it to hurt, I don't want it to be noticeable, and I don't want it to take very long. So what was the result of all of those combined treatments?

The results were my teeth were straightened and perfect within four months of beginning treatment. I was a minor case to begin with, and without the Acceledent and Propel, I would have estimated 12-15 months total. Those results were pretty good, I'd say! I would recommend the same to anyone who has the same concerns I had.

An added benefit for me getting my teeth straightened was being able to understand the process from a patient's point of view. For years, I would start treatment on patients and not see them for months at a time and it's really interesting to see what happens between those visits now. I am a much more empathetic and patient-conscious doctor. I have been through the same discomforts and embarrassments. I had a lot of the same concerns.

Sometimes orthodontic treatment can be uncomfortable. That's just a fact of treatment. We're moving teeth and bones around. Our goal is speed, convenience, discretion, and comfort. However, I can say, I do see the life changes that occur when a patient gets finished with treatment. I see the joy in a patient's eyes when he or she looks in the mirror. When comparing themselves with their pre-treatment photos, some will shed tears. It's awesome to be the architect of such change for the good. It's a really satisfying position for me to hold.

DR. MATTHEW R. WIRIG

SECTION 3

What Now? Questions and Answers for Your Treatment

DR. MATTHEW R. WIRIG

CHAPTER 11

How long does treatment take?

The length of treatment can depend on several factors. Minor problems can be corrected in a matter of a few weeks to months. More severe problems can take up to three years to correct. Most people wear braces from 12 to 18 months. The length of treatment also depends on several other important factors including:

Keeping and showing up for appointments

Not being able to show up for an appointment can slow down the progress of your child's treatments. Everyone understands there are emergencies which cannot be avoided. However, it is important to meet and keep regular appointments for your child's progress. Because many orthodontists have busy booking schedules, missing an appointment may set your child's treatment back since you will have to wait for the next available date to schedule a makeup appointment.

How often the brackets break

Broken brackets happen to just about every patient at least once or twice, but don't worry. It's a fairly common occurrence. A broken bracket doesn't necessarily mean that you (or your child) did anything wrong. When one of the brackets breaks, contact your orthodontist's office right away and ask for advice. Sometimes, they can fit your child in for an emergency appointment. Fortunately, Invisalign doesn't have brackets that can break, which is another reason why I recommend it.

Following the orthodontist's orders

You may be given special orders to wear rubber bands and other things. These can be uncomfortable at first, but they are there to help straighten the teeth. The more diligently you or your child follows the orthodontist's orders, the faster the process will go.

Whether your child's teeth are coming in

Once all the adult teeth have erupted and are coming in, it is easier for the orthodontist to straighten them. Healthy teeth can be straightened at any age, but the sooner the adult teeth are in, the easier it is for the orthodontist to straighten them. In rare and extreme cases, surgery may be needed to help bring the teeth in. These impactions are rare though, and we will only recommend surgery if we think it will really help.

Type of work needed

Each person and their case is unique. Orthodontists can only provide an estimated time and cannot guarantee anything. Be emotionally prepared for treatment to take slightly longer than the estimate.

When everything is done properly and treatment is not delayed due to breakages and poor compliance, is there any way to do it faster? The answer used to be no, but in the last five years, the answer is now yes. A new advancement in the world of orthodontics is accelerated tooth movement. Accelerating the process of orthodontic tooth movement is something new to those who want teeth moved quickly.

Accelerated orthodontics

Accelerated orthodontics is moving teeth faster than they would normally move during treatment. The accelerated methods have an added cost associated with them. However, they are gaining popularity for a variety of reasons, and speed is not the only reason!

They work by stimulating the bone and gums in the mouth in conjunction with Invisalign or braces. There are two main ways this is done.

Acceledent

Acceledent is a really cool, little, battery-powered device that is attached to a mouthpiece. Basically, it's a massager for your bite. But the massaging movements (also known as micropulses) and speed are drastically different than you would find in a commercial or home massaging device.

You wear the Acceledent device for 20 minutes a day. This is normally done at home while watching TV, checking email, or at other times you are not required to talk or move much. Users of Acceledent have noted less discomfort overall in their treatment as well as significantly faster treatment times. It can cut down on treatment time by as much as 30-40%!

Propel

Propel is a simple procedure done in office for patients. Propel is micro-perforations or tiny holes punched surgically into the bone around the teeth. Don't worry, it's perfectly safe. We wouldn't do it if it wasn't safe. This stimulates the bone to allow teeth to move faster.

The procedure, performed with anesthetic, is rather uneventful. Propel takes less than 30 minutes to perform. The worst part is getting numb and receiving the anesthesia. We use a strong topical gel that numbs the gums before we even anesthetize with a syringe of septocaine. Propel does cause some bruising of the soft tissue for a couple days, meaning your lips and gums in the areas where the perforations are made will be a little sore for a couple days.

We can only move teeth as fast as bone will allow, no matter what system of orthodontics is used (braces or Invisalign). When prescribed, some patients only need one treatment of Propel, while others will require multiple treatments spread out over multiple months. It really depends on the movements. I only had one treatment of Propel performed on me and it greatly enhanced the speed of movement of my teeth.

For someone who wants accelerated movement of teeth and shorter treatment times, I will almost always recommend Acceledent. I won't recommend Propel as often, but for some certain orthodontic movements, I will recommend it. When braces normally take two years, we can cut the time down tremendously using these treatments. Remember, I did both of these on my teeth when I did my Invisalign. It meant wearing Invisalign and being treated for months rather than years. What a tremendously awesome new enhancement to orthodontics.

DR. MATTHEW R. WIRIG

CHAPTER 12

How long are appointments?

Typical orthodontist appointments range anywhere from 15 minutes to an hour, with the average time being roughly 30 minutes long. If all you or your child needs is a basic exam, the appointment will go quicker. If your child needs his or her braces tightened or to have other adjustments done, the appointments can take longer. It is not common for an appointment to last longer than one hour. Putting on or removing braces takes about one hour to complete.

The first appointments for braces and Invisalign are very different.

When you get braces, the first appointment lasts about an hour to an hour and a half. This procedure is really painless for the most part. It doesn't hurt to put braces on, but it can be a little uncomfortable to have your mouth open for an hour. Other than having your mouth open for a little while, it's easy. Most people don't find it uncomfortable at all.

After signing a consent to treat and contract, the assistant will bring the doctor in with the patient to confirm the plan previously made and to answer any questions. At that time, the assistant will start to prepare the teeth to have the braces glued on. The assistant will need to have the doctor come in a couple of times during the process of bonding the braces. After the braces are bonded on, the assistant will put in a wire and have the patient choose colors for the braces. That's it!

The braces are on and ready to go. The last part of the appointment is to go over any questions and to teach you how to take care of the braces, as well as provide instructions on what can or cannot be eaten.

When you get braces, your appointments will usually be spaced out every 4-8 weeks for the duration of treatment. These appointments are usually short (20-30 minutes). These adjustment appointments allow us to modify the braces for how your teeth are moving and make any changes needed to get them perfect.

The final appointment to take braces off usually takes an hour. We do a lot during this appointment: we take the braces off, fit your bite for retainers, and take new sets of photos and x-rays for our records.

When you get Invisalign, the process is a little different, naturally. After deciding to start, you will have a 10-minute 3D scan taken of your teeth. But you will not be starting any treatment until your next appointment, which will be 2-3 weeks later.

At the next appointment, you will be given your first set of trays as well as having some tiny bumps of tooth colored material glued/bonded on your teeth. This takes about 30-45 minutes. You will be given several trays which you will use in a specific order. You will wear each tray for an average of two weeks, each. When you are done with one tray, you will discard it and move to the next tray.

We will only need to see you every 8-12 weeks after your first appointment. Each appointment, you will get a set of new trays to last you until your next appointment. You'll most likely need future scans and new sets of trays a couple of times during treatment. The first scan and first number of trays are not the end of your treatment. We will need to modify the movement of your teeth with each new scan to adjust for how your teeth respond to the Invisalign.

How long braces will remain on depends on multiple factors. The most important thing a patient can do to reduce the amount of time they need to wear braces is to follow the orthodontist's orders to the best of his or her ability.

Once it's time for the braces to come off, having the brackets removed does not hurt. You will feel a tugging and pulling sensation but that is about it. The orthodontist may need to scrape or polish any glue off of the teeth but it is not painful. The removal and cleaning up of the brackets takes about one hour.

DR. MATTHEW R. WIRIG

CHAPTER 13

How do I take care of my braces?

It is extremely important to understand how to take care of your teeth and braces. The basics are the same as taking care of your teeth normally. But the process is much more difficult at first, and if it's not done properly, bad things can happen to your teeth. Let's go over brushing first.

Use fluoride toothpaste or even a prescription fluoride toothpaste, and a soft, round-ended bristle toothbrush or power toothbrush that's in good condition.

Your regular manual toothbrush should be changed often. If you have a power toothbrush, the head should be changed often too. This is extremely important since the braces are really hard on the toothbrush and will wear out your bristles very quickly. The American Dental Association recommends replacing your brush or brush head about every three months. This means a new brush up to four times a year.

Brush around all the surfaces of your braces and every area or side of your teeth – fronts, sides, and backs, and on the top chewing surfaces for at least two full minutes, complete time. Many power toothbrushes are programmed to run for two minutes. It's important to brush your tongue and roof of the mouth as well.

A good way to tell if you're brushing enough and correctly is if your brackets are shiny and clean, and you cannot see any white film built up around or under them. Brush along your gum line gently and thoroughly. The area between the gum line and the braces is the most commonly missed and most important area to clean. It is in this area where you will develop decalcifications the quickest and worst. Decalcifications are the beginning of cavities forming. It is also removal in this area that prevents gingivitis from starting.

Rinse thoroughly with a mouthwash or water after you are done brushing. The best and most preferred mouth rinse to use is a fluoridated mouthwash, the most common is called ACT which is really easy to find at a drugstore.

Inspect your teeth and braces regularly. Make sure they are spotless from built up plaque or food. Look closely in the mirror. Every time you brush, it is a good time to check for loose/broken brackets and any other problems. If you find a problem, you should contact the orthodontist's office and see if it needs to be evaluated, and if you need to come into the office to have it repaired.

You should brush your teeth after every meal and often after every snack. If you can't brush right away, be sure to at least rinse your mouth out with water, swishing out any loose bits of food. It can be very helpful to carry a travel toothbrush with you to work or school, so that you can brush when not at home. At least once every day, you should clean between your teeth first with floss and then brush your teeth and brackets until they are thoroughly clean. The best time of the day to fully brush, floss, and rinse with a fluoride mouth rinse is at night, before you go to sleep.

Many children, teens, and even some adults don't know how to floss with braces on. Or they choose to avoid it because it can be more difficult than normal flossing. But daily flossing is especially important when you are wearing braces. This is because you're more likely to collect plaque in between your teeth. Food particles get trapped in the braces, bands, and wires. This can dramatically increase your risk of a cavity or gingivitis.

Be prepared to spend more time, as much as three times as long, on brushing and flossing when you have braces on your teeth. Although flossing with braces is not easy at first, you can get good at it with some practice. Here are some helpful tips for great flossing:

Use waxed floss (unwaxed floss will likely get caught in your braces and shred), dental tape, or a product like super floss.

Use enough floss; don't be frugal, floss is cheap. I recommend about 18 inches of floss, and in some cases, more.

Use a floss threader. A floss threader is much like a large sewing needle with a large eye to pass the floss through, only it's a really flimsy piece of plastic. You can tie the floss to the loop of the threader, which will then make it easier to thread the floss between and under wires.

Thread it carefully between teeth. Take the floss and carefully thread it under the main wire of the braces before passing it between two teeth with a flossing motion.

Then, when ready to move to the next spot, remove the floss and re-thread it under the main wire to pass between the next pair of teeth.

Be sure not to snap the floss simply up and down. You should gently wrap the floss against the side of each tooth, forming the shape of a C against each side of the teeth. Then draw the floss down under the gum tissue and back up, then do the other side between the same teeth the same way.

Some parents may need to do the flossing for younger children. This is needed when someone lacks the coordination to thread the floss under the main wire of his or her braces.

CHAPTER 14

What happens to your teeth if you do not brush?

Good brushing and flossing is critical during your orthodontic treatment. Without it, plaque and food can gather and build up around your braces. The bacteria in plaque react with sugars in the food you eat and form an acid that will dissolve away the enamel on your teeth. This can create a permanent white stain or mark on the teeth. These stains can be very noticeable and unsightly. The buildup of plaque can also cause cavities or gum disease.

1. The stains that are caused by the plaque around your braces are called **decalcifications**. Lines and spots from decalcification will stay on your teeth enamel for life, so the best way to avoid developing decalcification is to not let them develop at all. They can only be prevented with proper brushing and flossing daily.

2. Periodontal disease is caused by the buildup of plaque along the gum line and occurs in three stages. With the first stage, plaque deposits that are left along the gum line will irritate the gums. Your gums may become red, puffy, swollen, or enlarged. The gums will bleed when you brush and floss. The infection that is created by this is called **gingivitis**.

3. The second stage of periodontal disease progresses beyond gingivitis. If not corrected, infection and inflammation around and under the

97

gums will spread to the periodontal ligament and bone that surrounds and supports the teeth. The gums will start to separate from the teeth and fall away. This forms spaces or gaps called pockets between your teeth. This additional space allows more plaque to buildup and becomes harder to clean. This disease is called **periodontitis**.

4. The third stage of periodontal disease is the worst and hardest to fix. Pockets of bacteria will build up and form deeper beneath your gums. This attacks and eats away at the bone that holds your teeth in place and stabilizes them. This can cause your previously healthy teeth to loosen significantly, and eventually, they will need to be extracted. This disease is called **advanced periodontitis**.

What is Plaque?

Plaque is a white, hard to see, sticky film that builds up and collects on your teeth. It's composed primarily of bacteria, food bits, and saliva. When plaque and trapped foods/sugars are left on your braces or teeth, they will cause cavities, swollen gums, bad breath, and permanent white or brown stains on the surfaces of the teeth. Plaque builds up and can start to cause problems for your teeth within 24 hours. This is why the daily habit of removing it is so important. If plaque is left for long periods of time, it starts to harden and becomes what we call in dentistry, calculus. Calculus is much harder to clean off with normal brushing and flossing. The buildup of calculus is often the reason we are recommended to have a dental cleaning every six months. A dentist or dental hygienist has much better tools for removing calculus.

CHAPTER 15

What foods should I avoid?

This is the most common question I get during the time before a patient gets braces on. Obviously, parents are concerned about the management of their children's eating and want to avoid any possible harm to the investment made in braces.

The fact is, *you can still eat almost anything you want* when going through orthodontic treatment. We just want to avoid foods that can break brackets or ruin your braces. So generally, we want to avoid hard, chewy, or sticky foods, or foods that can get stuck between the teeth and gums.

There is no hard and fast list compiled somewhere with every food ever listed on it, and whether it's safe to eat or not. What I can do for you is provide you with some general guidelines that can help you understand what you should avoid. Good common sense should prevail when making decisions on what and what not to eat.

There are some foods that should be eaten carefully while having braces. Eating foods that are not compatible with braces can damage or dislodge the braces, and lead to a longer treatment time than was originally estimated. Here are a few guidelines to follow.

Hard foods should be avoided. Hard foods are commonly the reason for damage to braces. Here are a few examples of hard foods: Hard candies (i.e. Jolly Ranchers, jaw breakers, lollipops, Lemonheads), ice cubes, large nuts, and hard pretzels.

Hard foods can be eaten if they are first sliced into smaller pieces and chewed with your back teeth. These foods include fruits and vegetables, such as apples and carrots.

Chewy and sticky foods should be avoided. These foods will also easily dislodge the braces. Any food that requires a lot of effort to chew will usually damage the braces. Here are a few examples: Skittles, Starburst, Tootsie Rolls, caramel, jelly beans, taffy, beef jerky, Snickers, and bagels.

Softer foods that must be removed from harder surfaces should be eaten differently. The following foods are examples of what should be cut into small pieces (or removed from the bone or cob) before they are eaten: corn on the cob, spare ribs, and chicken wings.

Popcorn should be avoided. The problem with popcorn is parts of the kernel husk can become lodged between the teeth and gums. These remnants can be almost impossible for a patient to clean out when braces are present, and can lead to pain and inflammation of the gums.

Inedible items that are habitually chewed can easily damage the braces. Don't chew on pens, pencils, or finger nails.

You can eat and drink sugary foods and drinks. The problem isn't the sugar itself; the problem is making sure you keep your mouth clean after consuming the sugar. Sugar contributes to tooth decay and plaque formation.

Everyone is at risk of tooth decay from a diet high in sugar content. After drinking or eating sweet foods or drinks, it is important to brush your teeth. If it is impractical to brush at that time, it can help to at least rinse your mouth out thoroughly with water, swishing the water through your teeth. If you brush twice a day and floss once a day, and you make sure to swish with water or mouthwash after eating, you will be good to go!

Here are a few good examples of foods and drinks high in sugar content: milk, soda, coffee with cream, juice, doughnuts, candy, iced tea, chocolate, cereal, breath mints, cookies, cake, brownies.

Patients who wear Invisalign as an alternative to braces must be sure **not** to drink beverages with sugar or acids while wearing the aligners. The fluid can remain caught between the teeth and the aligners creating a breeding ground for bacteria. Aligners should be removed when drinking these types of things and the teeth rinsed or brushed whenever this happens.

SUGAR-FREE ALTERNATIVES ARE OKAY.

Some of these foods are also available in sugarless form, which is an acceptable alternative. In fact, I am a big proponent of patients chewing sugar-free gum. Sugar-free gum has been shown to have ingredients that actually fight against the bacteria that form plaque in the mouth, and some have a molecule known to re-mineralize teeth. Sugar-free gum has also been known to bring comfort to some patients, when they chew, suffering from the tooth pain that orthodontics cause. The chewing pressures can soothe the achy teeth.

Xylitol is a sweetener often used in sugar-free gum. It's very good for teeth as it interferes with the growth and reproduction of bacteria. Sugarless gum also removes bacteria when you chew it, which helps to clean your mouth. Chewing sugarless gum for 1-10 minutes after eating is good for your teeth.

CHAPTER 16

How to handle Orthodontic Emergencies

In this section, I am going to share with you the most common orthodontic emergencies as they apply to braces. I am going to list them in order from least severe to most severe. One of the benefits of Invisalign is most of these emergencies do not apply to Invisalign treatment and the amount of things that could go wrong is significantly less when being treated with Invisalign.

Remember, these are listed in least to greatest severity. Only the most severe problem needs to be seen immediately by an orthodontist or one of his or her staff members. The majority of these smaller problems can be addressed at the patient's next scheduled appointment. Orthodontic offices are equipped to instruct patients on the urgency of a specific problem. Remember, orthodontic movement of teeth is a slow process that takes time. It is rare that something would ever be urgent and require immediate attention. Just give your office a call and ask, if you have any questions.

Food Caught Between Teeth

Having food caught in your braces and between teeth is inevitable for every patient. This is not a true emergency, but can be annoying and frustrating to deal with until you have learned how to manage it. It can be both uncomfortable and embarrassing to have food caught in between teeth and in the braces. Effective use of floss and using a good flossing technique is effective in fixing this problem. Other devices that may help in these cases are floss threaders, orthodontic/braces specific flossers, super floss, interproximal brushes, and toothpicks, which can be effective in helping solve this problem. Instead of saving your dinner in your braces for later, clean it out and smile more comfortably and confidently.

Ligatures Come Off

The word ligature means the little colored rubber bands or small fine wires that hold the wire into the individual brackets. It takes a finely skilled hand to place the colored rubber bands on the braces as well as a good, sterile pair of tweezers. If, instead of a rubber band, a small fine wire is tied around the brace and an end is poking out, use the end of a pencil with its eraser to push the wire out of the way and so that it is not poking anymore.

Of course, if either comes loose or is lost, it may need to be replaced; feel free to call your orthodontist and inquire about the issue. A staff member should be able to tell you if it needs to be seen soon or if it can wait till your next appointment.

Bite Feels Strange or Teeth Feel Loose

It is a completely normal thing for patients to become frustrated with how their bite works or doesn't work anymore while in the middle of treatment. When I did my Invisalign treatment, I was frustrated that my teeth did not function the same way as they did prior to treatment. One of the reasons for this was that my bite was not perfect. I was used to functioning with a bad bite. So, that takes some getting used to.

At one point, as my teeth were moving, my front teeth couldn't touch when I tried to bite down. As it was changing, I was also frustrated that some teeth felt loose or tender as well. I couldn't bite through that tough piece of beef jerky anymore with my front teeth. Then a few weeks later, I was able to bite with my front teeth, but my back teeth didn't work together quite right and I had the opposite problem. The reality is that we are creatures of habit and get used to doing things a certain way. During treatment, teeth are moving and the bite is changing. It may take time to get used to the changes. In fact, things may seem worse or seem as though they are not getting better. Don't worry, your smile and bite will be better after treatment is completed.

We often advise patients who are concerned about this. Sometimes it may get or look worse before it gets better. This is perfectly normal. Orthodontists are highly trained in what we do. Just leave it to me and my trusted team of skilled professionals. We will get you the results you want if you follow the course of treatment to the end.

Think of it similarly to repainting your car. The first step is to remove the previous paint and/or put a coat of primer on. If you were to judge the paint job at this point, it would not be fair. The priming is necessary for a good result in the end. However, at that point, it does not look good. The point at which you should judge the paint job is when it is completed. This is the ideal time to judge the results.

Spaces appear in places they never have before

When we begin orthodontic treatment, sometimes we will create spaces in places where they never existed before. This can be most frustrating if it happens in between the two front teeth. This is a normal part of braces for some people. It is not an indication of the final results, and although frustrating, it does mean progress is being made. Be assured that as easily as the space opens up, it is just as easy to close it. Sometimes we will wait to close the space; this may be necessary so that it is closed correctly and with good results.

Consult with your orthodontist if you have concerns like this. He or she will be able to explain the process and plan for your specific case.

Discomfort

It is normal to have discomfort for a day or two after an adjustment of the braces or when putting in a new Invisalign aligner. The teeth themselves may become tender to the touch and experience sensitivity to hot and cold, temporarily.

Any discomfort that is lingering and does not subside in a few days to a couple of weeks should be discussed with your orthodontist. Softer foods are a way to avoid some of the discomfort as well as rinsing with warm salt water. Over-the-counter pain medications can be very helpful as well, these would include acetaminophen (Tylenol) and ibuprofen (Motrin/Advil). There have been some really good studies that show a significant decrease in pain when these are used. The best results are often seen using ibuprofen. Just take the recommended amount for your age and size, as instructed on the bottle.

Most orthodontists like myself don't have the legal ability to prescribe medications. The strongest thing we would ever recommend would be over-the-counter ibuprofen. This can be obtained at any drug store, pharmacy, and many other places.

Irritation of Lips or Cheeks

The mouth is a really incredibly tough place. When you think about it, we are pouring really strong acids into our mouths with sour candies, hot sauces, and soda. We pour scalding hot and freezing cold liquids into our mouths. We also mash up crunchy foods and some of us crush ice in our mouths (by the way, chewing ice is not good). I'm amazed we don't cause far more damage to our mouths and teeth than we already do.

Almost everyone has been a victim of a canker sore on the lip. Who hasn't burned themselves by drinking hot cocoa/coffee? Or tore up the roof of their mouth on some cereal? It's not terribly uncommon for your mouth to develop little sores from the braces or Invisalign trays as well.

I was a victim of an Invisalign tray constantly irritating the side of my tongue. Or if I slept on my stomach, my face and cheek would become pressed into the side of the Invisalign edge. Or I would find my tongue playing with the edge of the tray, and then I would get a sore on my tongue from the habit. It is inevitable. Our mouths will find ways to be annoyed by what we put in it. So, this shouldn't come as a surprise. I can tell you it will all go away with time.

Your body will adapt to the annoyance and it will get better on its own most of the time.

If, however, you can remove the irritation without damaging the appliances, then it can speed up the process. We give every patient who gets braces a little package of wax. Wax can be useful when applying to the offending area on the braces or Invisalign. When it is put on repeatedly, it allows the area to heal up. When the offended area is healed, it is less likely to be damaged again. The mouth is similar to our hands. When working in a garden or with hand tools, your hands will toughen up and develop calluses that protect them from the rigors of the work. Our mouths will toughen up in the same way. This means you should only rely on wax when you have an open sore which has developed and not for other minor annoyances. You should be able to wean yourself off of wax and only need use of it occasionally.

A small amount of relief wax can be an excellent buffer between the braces and your cheeks. Simply pinch off a small piece and roll it into the size of a small pea. As best as you can, dry off the area on your braces where you intend to apply it. Then, flatten the small ball of wax over the dried area on your braces. You will then be able to eat more comfortably and the area will heal easier. Everything in the mouth takes only a few days to heal, although some sores take up to two weeks. If you accidentally swallow or eat the wax, it is ok. The wax will not hurt you if ingested. It is harmless.

With Invisalign, we have the added advantage of being able to trim the aligner so that the offending edge does not cause the same irritation. I often instruct my Invisalign patients to use sterile, disinfected fingernail clippers to clip off an edge that is causing a sore. It's a fast and easy fix for patients with Invisalign. Don't clip off too much though!

Check with your orthodontist before making any major modifications to your aligners. Wax can be used to great effect with Invisalign as well, although we see far less irritation in the mouth from patients using Invisalign.

Protruding wire

When you start wearing braces, the wires zig and zag in and out in order to conform to a patient's crooked teeth. As the teeth straighten, the wire itself does not need to bend as much. When this happens, the wire will start to creep out the back of the braces and become extended. When a wire is protruding out of the back of the braces, it can sometimes be irritating because it may catch the cheek or embed itself in the gums. The good thing about this is it is an indication of progress; the teeth are moving and getting straighter. The bad thing is, of course, it can be uncomfortable.

At other times, the wire may protrude from different circumstances. When this happens, it may need to be clipped by the office staff or be seen by the orthodontist. Notify the office if it cannot be resolved by methods discussed previously.

Those methods mentioned previously involve using a pencil eraser to move the wire, or a pair of tweezers to reinsert it into a brace, or placing wax to temporarily solve the problem. If the situation is extremely bothersome and it is impractical to be seen soon for an appointment, you may try clipping the wire yourself with sterile/disinfected nail clippers.

The main thing to be careful of is to not allow the clipped wire to be swallowed or lost after clipping! This can be helped by using gauze or cotton balls to stabilize the wire while it is being cut. This can be scary to do, and you don't want to break the wire, so call your orthodontist if you have questions.

You can avoid this issue with Invisalign. For most patients, the protruding wire is not noticeable nor a problem, as it is usually trimmed and accounted for at each appointment.

Loose Brackets, Wires, Bands, or Attachments

If any fixed part of the braces such as a bracket, wire, band, or in the case of attachments on Invisalign, come loose, or break off, you should notify the orthodontic office. This is especially important if you were just seen recently for an appointment and don't have an appointment for a while. Broken or loose parts can mean longer overall treatment times. The faster something is fixed, the better your treatment will stay on track. If your appointment is coming up soon, it would still be good to let us know beforehand what is possibly wrong, but we may advise you to be seen at your regular appointment.

The average patient breaks two brackets during the entire course of his or her treatment. This is normal and unavoidable because our mouths are such active places. Multiple things can cause excessive breakage of brackets. The rarest cause is improper bonding technique or faulty materials. This does happen, but for most orthodontists, it is extremely rare. The most common cause of breakage is careless management of the braces or improper diet – eating foods that will break the braces. Certain types of bites can also cause breakages. Some people with strong jaw muscles or deep bites are more prone to having braces break off. Another cause may be malformed enamel. Enamel is the hard outer layer of teeth. At times, it may form in an abnormal way and may be difficult for the braces' adhesives/glues to work.

A really conscientious patient who follows the rules and is careful will have the fewest problems and the fastest treatment times.

Piece of Appliance is swallowed

With so much in the mouth and so much on the teeth with braces, sometimes, as much as we work to avoid it, something may come loose and get swallowed. This is rare, but when it does happen, it can be fairly alarming to the patient. If something is swallowed, most of the time it is harmless. The most common thing swallowed is wax or rubber bands. Neither of these things will cause a problem. Most other things will not cause a problem either. If you are worried about having swallowed anything, you should contact your orthodontist's office.

Most of these events are not even true emergencies. The true orthodontic emergency is really very rare. It would only be considered a true emergency if it is required to be sent to an emergency room. This is most often the case when someone has had a severe accident and has broken teeth and/or the jawbones. In these cases, it is much more important to be seen by a general dentist, physician, and/or oral surgeon before being seen by an orthodontist.

One of the advantages to wearing braces or Invisalign is that if there is a true emergency and some damage has been done to the teeth or jaw, the amount of damage caused is often severely lessened by wearing braces. Meaning, it is much harder to get a tooth knocked out when wearing braces or Invisalign. It is still a good idea to wear athletic mouth guards while wearing braces. If nothing else, it will prevent your cheeks from getting torn up by the braces if you get an impact to the face.

I recently saw a patient who came in after being hit with a baseball at a practice. The baseball had dislodged his tooth and it was only being held in by the braces themselves. He was really fortunate because the bone was damaged around the front teeth also and was broken. Because he was wearing braces, everything was stabilized and not falling out. This sounds rather gruesome, but he was pretty fortunate.

The advantage of Invisalign when someone receives trauma is that it serves much in the same way as mouth guard and protects the mouth and teeth.

CHAPTER 17

Frequently asked questions about orthodontics

Do braces hurt?

Most people experience varying amounts of pain when having treatment. It's really hard to tell you how much you will have, individually. Women are more tolerant to pain than men. Children are more tolerant to pain than adults. Smokers feel more pain than non-smokers.

Studies have shown that patients with Invisalign experience less pain, as do patients who use Acceladent. There are different types of pain. Tooth pain (or an ache) is experienced with any tooth movement usually for about 3-5 days, but varies greatly due to the individual. Soft tissue (gums) pain can occur when braces or Invisalign cause trauma to the lips and gums. Braces create soft tissue (gums) trauma more often, but the mouth and lips toughen up. It gets better, the longer you have braces on.

I recently put braces on my oldest child, Brooklynn.

Allow me to brag about her just a little bit. One day when I was struggling to put together a trampoline for her and her siblings, she took notice. I hadn't followed directions as closely as I should have and was having to take it apart multiple times and reassemble it. I was sweating profusely, and she disappeared and returned a few minutes later with a big glass of ice water. She said, "Daddy, I saw you might need a drink!" Nothing humbles you as fast a random act of kindness like that. I felt bad for losing my patience a couple times while assembling the trampoline.

She's a sweet girl and she always seems to be looking for ways to help out.

As a side note to that story, read the directions closely when assembling a trampoline, and even the small steps and directions are important to follow. This is the same with orthodontic treatment: <u>Follow the advice and recommendations we give you. If you do, you will have less pain, faster treatment, and better results!</u>

The day I put braces on Brooklynn, we were both so excited. I put them on her in the morning, and my wife took her home. When I got home from work, I found her straight away and asked her what she thought. But the glow in her eyes was gone. Almost in tears she said, "Daddy, they hurt." It broke my heart to know I was inflicting pain on my child.

The next day, I asked Brooklynn if she was still in pain. To my relief, she hasn't complained about them since. Luckily, this is the experience most children have. Although some may have it for more than a day.

Are shots necessary?

No, shots are not a normal part of orthodontic treatment for most patients. In the rare circumstance that you are prescribed Temporary Anchorage Devices or Propel Accelerated Orthodontics, then minor anesthesia may be required.

Will I need permanent teeth extracted?

Each person's teeth and problems are unique to themselves. Some patients require teeth to be extracted and some do not. The decision to extract any teeth should be taken very seriously and only be done if absolutely necessary. Orthodontists try to avoid extracting teeth if they can, but at times, it is the right thing to do.

In my personal practice, we are very conservative and lean toward less extractions overall. But if, by not extracting, it will create more problems with the teeth and make the teeth less healthy or less stable, then it's in the best interest of patients to have some teeth extracted. I only recommend extracting or any treatments for that matter that I would perform on my own family members or children too, if they had the same problems. In fact, when doing an exam, I often ask myself, "If this were one of my children, what would I recommend?"

For severe cases of crowding, jaw discrepancy, or to achieve good facial balance, some tooth extraction may be required.

What are Temporary Anchorage Devices? Mini-Implants/TADs?

These terms all relate to a miniature titanium implant that can be placed during an appointment through the gum tissue and into the bone of a patient. It's a relatively simple and quick procedure. TADs are used to assist in dramatic movement of teeth that would otherwise be unachievable.

They can help prevent the need for more complicated surgeries. You may require local anesthesia/numbing to have the TAD inserted. They are generally painless after placement and are easily removed after treatment. They are only placed temporarily and removed when no longer needed.

Do I still need to visit the dentist while in braces?

Absolutely. As orthodontists, we are limited to offering only orthodontic treatment. Of course, I am constantly inspecting visually for anything of concern. If I see signs of something specifically going on which requires dental attention, I'll encourage you to speak to your dentist.

We do not take the necessary, close up x-rays which show developing cavities. So it is important to have that monitored, especially when you have braces on. We advise every patient on the necessity of seeking regular dental care. It is a prerequisite for being treated, and we will discontinue treatment if patients are not seeing their dentist regularly. Orthodontics is great and straighter teeth are wonderful, but the overall health of a patient, including the health of his or her teeth is more important than the benefits of braces. If you have no teeth, then it won't matter if they are straight.

How do I get my teeth cleaned with braces on?

It is important to maintain your regular appointments for teeth cleanings. The standard recommendation is six months, and some people need them more frequently than this. Some dentists or hygienists clean your teeth without having wires removed for the cleaning. Some require the wires to be removed. If the wire is not to be removed, then make your appointment with the dentist office like you would normally. But it is easier for the hygienist to clean the teeth with the wire removed; however, this will involve more appointments to do so. If you need the wire removed, you will need to make an appointment with your orthodontist to remove the wire the day before or on the same day as the cleaning appointment. Then you will need to have the wire replaced, either immediately following the appointment or the next day. This will ensure there is no interruption in the treatment progress.

Will wisdom teeth mess up my bite and make my teeth crowded?

This is possibly the biggest misconception in all of orthodontics, and it drives me nuts!

Many people and even dental professionals are out of the loop on the current research and are still telling patients that wisdom teeth are the cause of teeth crowding. There has been extensive research done on this, and we have learned that whether you have wisdom teeth or not, your teeth will crowd over time, especially the ones on the bottom front.

Your teeth will crowd whether you get your wisdom teeth out or not. I don't want to minimize the need to get wisdom teeth out. There are still a ton of reasons to have them removed. Wisdom teeth can be and should be extracted at an optimal time for the procedure. Wisdom teeth cause enough other problems that we generally recommend they be extracted from most people.

Regardless of having wisdom teeth removed or not, wearing retainers is extremely important. It is something you have to commit to wearing for the rest of your life, at least at nights while sleeping.

When did orthodontics begin?

In America, orthodontics made its first appearance more than a hundred years ago. In 1880, Dr. Edward Angle pioneered a system of categorizing dental irregularities. And in 1900, he founded the first dental specialty organization, now known as the American Association of Orthodontists. Today, the AAO has more than 8,500 active, practicing members in the U.S. and Canada, and more than 13,500 members worldwide.

What is a 5-Star Patient?

We are so glad to be chosen by our patients for their orthodontic treatment. Our goal is to be a 5-star practice for our patients. Our favorite way of getting new patients is by referrals from current patients. Rather than giving money to an advertising company, we'd rather have lots of fun and cool rewards for patients who refer us to their friends and family!

We are a referral-based business and we ask our patients to help build our practice. In return, we offer great perks and rewards for doing things to help promote our practice. We have identified some practice-building tasks that really benefit our practice, and we reward our patients with cool prizes when they complete those tasks for us. These practice-building tasks include things like Facebook reviews and likes, online reviews, written testimonials, video testimonials, and patients referring their friends and families. We even give our patients a rating based on the number of positive referrals/feedback/reviews they have done for us, and we reward our patients when they achieve 5 stars.

Rewards range from a chance to spin the wheel of fun to a personalized thank-you from the doctor himself, and we are even giving away a car to one lucky patient! We are always looking for new, exciting, and fun ways to reward our patients. Our goal is to give you an experience like no other.

DR. MATTHEW R. WIRIG

SECTION 4

What happens after braces?

CHAPTER 18

Retainers

After wearing braces for a period of time, we will remove them and you (or your child) will have the smile you always wanted. No more brackets, wires, or bands, and you will be able to brush and floss easily. You will feel the smoothness of your tooth enamel on your cheeks and tongue.

Even though your active treatment is over and this is a new day, remember, you are starting a new phase of treatment. This phase is called the retention phase.

The retention phase of treatment is just as important as the active phase. Even though your teeth are straight, they will not stay that way without some form of retention. Why go through the process of treatment in the first place if you can't keep the results?

Retention involves wearing a custom-made appliance called a retainer. Several different types of retainers are available, with numerous variations of each type. We will give you recommendations and instructions on how to wear retainers and how long to keep them on.

Teeth are not held solidly in place in the jaw. They are floating inside the jaw instead. Held in place by a group of stretchy fibers called the periodontal ligament. After teeth and the periodontal ligament have being moved, it takes a number of months for the bone and the periodontal ligament to readjust to the new tooth position. So, if you want to keep those straight teeth and great smile, you must wear a retainer. Straightening teeth takes a lot of time, effort, and money to get great results; retainers are a small price to pay to ensure the investment is lasting.

The very day you get the braces off, you will be fitted for retainers. This is the perfect time because your teeth are at their most perfect point at this moment. We first remove the braces, and then we polish your teeth. Once the braces are off and the teeth are free, we take final x-rays and photos for our records. Then, we'll take impressions for retainers and start to get them ready.

There are three basic types of retainers available today; each works differently and there is no perfect solution or retainer. The most recognizable is the Hawley retainer. This is a piece of acrylic that is molded to the inside, tongue-side of your teeth, with a wire that wraps around the cheek-side of your teeth. The Hawley retainer can be made or personalized with multiple colors and designs; it is simple, durable, and easy to remove. It can be adjusted for some minor movements. Its biggest disadvantage is that it costs a little more to make because it is put together by a dental lab, and it can't be made the same day. It often takes a couple of days or a week to receive your retainer.

An increasing popular type of retainer is the clear aligner essix type, which looks similar to the Invisalign® system. These practically invisible retainers are custom-made of transparent plastic that fits securely over your teeth, covering them completely. Their main advantage is they are less expensive overall, quick to make, and they are clear. The essix retainers are easy to remove, but they may be a little less durable than the Hawley, long-term. They do allow you to perform whitening procedures with them. This is the type of retainer preferred by most patients, and the type that we provide for our patients. In fact, we provide two sets of them because a backup retainer is a wonderful thing in this world of retainer-eating dogs and careless teenagers.

The third type of retainer is the fixed retainer. It is preferred by some people, especially on the lower front teeth. Being fixed means it isn't removable to brush and floss your teeth. This retainer is a wire that is glued or bonded to the back-side of the teeth, where your tongue touches. It may remain in place for months, years, or longer. This type of retainer is used for rare cases when the teeth will not stay straight from another type of retainer. The main disadvantage of this type of retainer is it is really hard to keep the teeth clean under the wire. This means patients have to be extremely diligent about brushing and flossing, as well as seeing their dentist for routine cleanings and checkups.

With any major change, it takes time to adjust to something new. People are creatures of habit and generally dislike change. Retainers feel different when compared to braces or Invisalign. With time most people adjust really well to wearing retainers on a consistent and regular basis. It may stimulate your mouth to create more saliva, and it may be difficult to speak properly at first, but those changes will disappear with time. You may take them out to brush your teeth or eat.

In most cases, you will be instructed to wear your retainer at nights only. However, some patients will be instructed to wear their retainers more often. It is important to follow the instructions of your orthodontist when wearing retainers.

Caring for your retainer

Retainers come with a couple of strict rules. The first one is to store your retainer in its case when it is not being worn. This makes it hard to lose and easy to find. Never place your retainer in a place where pets can get to them. They are notorious for being chew toys for dogs. You should clean your retainer daily with a toothbrush and a splash of mouthwash.

There are two common ways I often hear about patients losing a retainer. One is to have a dog chew it up. The other is to throw it away at a restaurant by wrapping it in a napkin and not keeping it in the case.

To stay clean and fresh, all retainers need proper cleaning in order to remove germs. A Hawley retainer can be brushed gently with a regular toothbrush and toothpaste. However, toothpaste may scratch the clear aligner types. Denture cleaners sold at drugstores come in a powder or tablet form and can be used to clean and disinfect most removable retainers. Recently, the same cleaners have been packaged as retainer cleaners. They are the same thing, just marketed specifically for retainers.

Fixed non-removable retainers are cleaned by brushing and flossing your teeth. Cleaning is similar to maintaining braces, and you may need a floss threader or interproximal brush to serve as a tool to clean around and under the wire.

If you always remember to use the retainer case for storage, your chances of losing the retainer are greatly decreased. You should never boil your retainer or clean it in the dishwasher. Heat can warp and bend the retainer, so be careful not to lay it next to a curling iron or hair dryer. If it becomes warped, it will become unusable. With proper care and conscientiousness, a retainer can last for a long time and will help your smile last for a longtime.

How long do you wear a retainer?

Retainers are required for as long as you want your teeth to remain straight. It is true that the teeth are most vulnerable to relapse in the months immediately after having the braces removed; however, this is not the only time they will move. Orthodontists used to recommend, generally, that people wear retainers full-time for a year. Immediately after ceasing retainer wear, teeth stayed relatively stable for most people, but as people aged, things changed. Those same people now have shifted teeth and many are getting braces again for a second time.

The most common times that patients' teeth move is when the body is undergoing a lot of changes. It's no wonder that it is very common for teeth to shift for women when they are pregnant. Like in the case of my wife. She had braces when she was younger. However, when she failed to wear her retainer when she was pregnant with our first child, her teeth shifted. She wanted to straighten her teeth after she was done having children to make up for the changes that occurred.

Since we know we have to wear retainers forever now, we have most patients wear them only at nights from the start. We want to create great habits from the get-go. Another advantage of clear tray type retainers is, if they are worn forever, they will protect the teeth from grinding. This protection will benefit your teeth in the long-term. You may have to replace the retainers every now and again, but you won't have to replace your teeth.

CHAPTER 19

What do I do if I (or my child) has an
accident and breaks a tooth?

Preventing accidents is the easiest way to deal with them, but we cannot prevent them all. You should have some basic understanding of how to handle them and who to contact in the event of an accident.

Mouth guards are one of the easiest and least expensive ways to avoid tooth damage. They help minimize and prevent injuries to the teeth, jaws, and brain. The American Association of Orthodontists recommends mouth guards be worn whenever someone could come into contact with a ball, a hard object, another player, or the pavement. The recommendation applies to organized sports as well as other activities like skateboarding or cycling. If a mouth guard is not worn and an injury occurs, here are some simple tips.

Broken Tooth

If you encounter a broken tooth, you should carefully clean the area, apply an ice pack for any swelling, and keep the broken part of the tooth, if possible, in some type of container. Then promptly call your general dentist and have the broken tooth evaluated. You may be able to have the broken part reattached to the tooth.

Loose or Displaced Tooth

A loose or displaced tooth will either be really wiggly and or appear as if the tooth has moved instantly to a new position. It can appear to have moved higher, lower, or to the side. The first step would be to gently try to move it back. If it does not move with gentle force, do not attempt to move with heavier force. Then apply an ice pack and make arrangements to see your general dentist.

Knocked-Out Tooth

When a tooth is knocked out, time is critical. It is important to seek treatment as soon as possible. Call your general dentist or pediatric dentist immediately. It is important to gently handle the tooth by the crown. This is the part that is widest, and not the thinner pointed end. You can quickly rinse off any large debris or other dirt. Do not scrub the tooth, just gently rinse it. Then you can try to place it back into the socket.

If it does go back into the socket, then hold it in place until you are seen by a dentist. If it cannot be placed back into the socket, then it needs to be stored carefully. It is important the tooth doesn't dry out, but it is also important to not use water to store it in. The only readily available liquids good for storage of a knocked-out tooth are: milk, contact lens saline solution (without preservatives), and the saliva of the person who had it knocked out.

Here is another alternative. Just tuck it in your cheek, being careful not to swallow it, and seek dental treatment as soon as possible from your general dentist. If you cannot get to a dentist within a few hours, you can keep it in your cheek until you are able to get it into one of the above mentioned solutions.

DR. MATTHEW R. WIRIG

CHAPTER 20

When can I get my teeth whitened?

Who doesn't want whiter teeth? Everybody loves a smile that is bright and white. There are many products and procedures available to improve the look of your smile and make your teeth look whiter. We often get patients wanting to whiten their teeth after braces or Invisalign. Let's discuss the different options.

There are three types of whitening treatments available to consumers:

Professionally Supervised Treatment

The first is offered by dental professionals and sold through their offices. Professional teeth whitening by your dentist or orthodontist is the best choice when you want or need immediate whitening results. This procedure can be done chair-side in the office or can be done as take-home option.

These treatments prescribed by your dentist or orthodontist are generally stronger and require more supervision. If you obtain the bleaching solutions from your doctor's office, we will make a custom-fitting, whitening tray that will fit very securely to your teeth. The advantage to a custom tray is you are less likely to have irritations on the gum tissue when bleaching.

Home Whitening Treatment

The second type of treatment is over-the-counter treatments sold in drugstores and other retailers. These tend to be less powerful and more diluted gels when compared to professional whitening. They can get your teeth white, but it may take longer and require significantly more treatments. The other disadvantage is the mouthpieces are not custom fit to your teeth.

There are many different ways to deliver the whitening because it has been hard to find a system as effective as a custom-made tray. Some systems are paint-on systems, while some are strips of thin film covered in bleach. However, the most common involves a simple mouthpiece.

The teeth-whitening procedures can have minor side effects. When you have a bothersome side effect, you should speak with your dentist. For example, tooth and gum tissue can become sensitive or irritated during the period when you are using the bleaching solution. This sensitivity, in most cases, is temporary. The sensitivity should lessen once the treatment is finished.

Whitening Toothpaste

The third way to whiten teeth is also the least effective. These are whitening toothpastes. Personally, I have not noticed any difference visually from the usage of these whitening toothpastes for me or any patient.

There is some science behind it. All toothpastes help remove stains on the surface of your teeth. It does this through the action of mild abrasive particles in the toothpastes. Whitening toothpastes have an additional substance/chemical agent which provides more effective stain removal. Unlike bleaching treatments, these toothpastes do not alter the natural color of teeth, they just scrub them and lift off stains better. They likely work better with patients who drink a lot of coffee, tea, wine, or those who smoke. Substances that stain the teeth are more easily removed with these toothpastes.

When using whitening toothpastes, know that it's these abrasives in the toothpaste that can also scratch your clear retainers or Invisalign aligners. So, don't use this kind of toothpaste to clean them.

CHAPTER 21

Answers to other questions you may have

Will my child be able to return to school the same day he/she receives braces?

Often when we are putting braces on children, I will recommend that they return to school for the day. The thing about orthodontic discomfort is that it is always worse when someone is sitting around bored, watching TV, or doing something else that doesn't require much thought. It is so much better to go back to school and be forced to stay busy. You will think about your teeth so much less. Plus, since braces are cool nowadays, unlike when I was a child, kids should get to work showing them off to their friends!

Can

Absolutely! As with all individuals, we recommend wearing a mouth guard to protect the face, teeth, mouth, and brain from impact. Many kids play football or wrestle with braces; pretty much any sport is going to work out fine.

Can I still play musical instruments with braces?

Playing a wind instrument is a complex task involving the muscles of the face and lips, the tongue and the teeth. Some musicians who play a wind instrument may find that orthodontic treatment affects their ability to practice and perform. Inexperienced musicians will probably find that wearing braces doesn't change their performance very much, but more experienced, proficient players may notice a greater change. The good news is, that with practice and motivation, most wind instrument players can adjust to wearing braces.

Invisalign can make it a non-issue.

What is root resorption?

Root resorption is a shortening of the roots during orthodontics. It is a rare thing to have damage to the roots from treatment but it can occur. In a few patients, it can be seen as nothing more than a slight roundedness of the root tips. This generally will not result in any long-term problems for those teeth. An even rarer situation will develop in some patients where up to one-half or more of the root shortens away. This could affect the long-term health and stability of those affected teeth. The exact cause is not completely known at this time, and there is no effective way of predicting if it will occur. Although, it is known that braces over a long period of time (i.e. over 2-3 years) will increase the chances of root resorption. Many orthodontists will take initial, mid-treatment, and final panoramic x-rays to determine if root resorption has occurred during treatment.

DR. MATTHEW R. WIRIG

CHAPTER 22

Conclusion

An orthodontic professional can help you greatly improve your smile and teeth for years to come. You have a variety of treatment options to consider. While it may seem overwhelming for you to consider, I hope that I have left you with some food for thought. Rest assured in knowing that orthodontic treatment is far beyond what it was in past generations. We can do some pretty great things with the help of modern orthodontic technology.

When you come to see us at Wirig Orthodontics, we will do our best to answer any other questions you may have. We are here for you and we want to make the process as seamless and enjoyable as possible. We want to serve you "PIE" by Positively Impacting Everyone.

Consider the long-lasting benefits that go along with straightening teeth. As I spoke about in the book, it changes lives.

Lastly, consider this: Our initial consultations are FREE. There's no risk or cost for you to sit down with me or one of my doctors and discuss you and/or your child's case.

You can setup your FREE exam and X-Rays ($300 value) at our Henderson or Las Vegas locations by calling 702-454-1008! I hope to see you soon.

ABOUT THE AUTHOR

Dr. Wirig is an orthodontic specialist (NV S3-175) who currently practices in Henderson and Las Vegas, Nevada. He graduated cum laude in 2006 from UNLV's School of Dental Medicine and then finished a two-year orthodontic residency at UNLV in 2008. He owns and operates two orthodontic practices and employs several associate orthodontists. He is the Past-President of the Nevada Orthodontic Society (2012-2014). He has earned numerous awards, distinctions, and recognitions for his academic and clinical work. He is a member of Omicron Kappa Upsilon Dental Honor Society and the American Association of Orthodontics. Dr. Wirig is actively involved in civic, professional, and religious activities in Clark County, Nevada. In 2014, Dr. Wirig took a faculty position at UNLV's Orthodontic Residency Program, where he teaches dental residents who will become future orthodontists.

You can set up your FREE exam and X-Rays ($300 value) at our Henderson or Las Vegas locations by calling (702) 848-4585!

Get your free Orthodontic Decision-Making Kit! Just go to http://UltimateSmileGuide.com. Your kit includes:

- Our report, "The Caring Parent's Guide To Orthodontics: Five Factors To Know Before Getting Braces or Invisalign"

- A downloadable recording of Dr. Wirig on Business Innovators Radio called "Specialization and Technology: How To Get The Fastest, Most Comfortable Orthodontic Treatment Available"

- A digital copy of this book

Go to http://UltimateSmileGuide.com